The UNIQUE PRINCIPLE:
The Philosophy *of* MACROBIOTICS

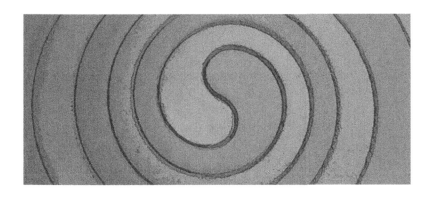

GEORGE OHSAWA

George Ohsawa Macrobiotic Foundation
Chico, California
www.ohsawamacrobiotics.com

Other Books by George Ohsawa
Book of Judo
Cancer and the Philosophy of the Far East
Essential Ohsawa
Gandhi, the Eternal Youth
Macrobiotic Guidebook for Living
Macrobiotics: An Invitation to Health and Happiness
Macrobiotics: The Way of Healing
Order of the Universe
Philosophy of Oriental Medicine
Practical Guide to Far Eastern Macrobiotic Medicine
Zen Macrobiotics

Unique Principle was originally published in French by J. Vrin Philosophical Library in Paris in 1931. It is George Ohsawa's first book and is thus very important to understanding his unique philosophy. The English edition was edited by Herman Aihara.

With appreciation—Robert Nissenbaum

Cover design by Carl Campbell
Text layout and design by Carl Ferré

First English Edition	1973
Current Edition: edited and reformatted	2010 Dec 7

Published with the help of East West Center for Macrobiotics
    www.eastwestmacrobiotics.com

ISBN 978-0-918860-17-0

Preface to the English Edition

This book is unique, not because of its name or its contents, but rather how it was translated and published. The translation of this book was started by a group of macrobiotic practitioners in Chico, California about seven years ago. Lou Oles, one of the group, then moved to Los Angeles and continued the translation.

After Lou Oles died in 1967, the work moved to Boston, where I am uncertain how many people worked on the book's translation and revision. Strangely, however, on one day this year, I found the completed translation on my desk at George Ohsawa Macrobiotic Foundation in San Francisco. I started plans to publish it right away. Thus, the translation of this book was completed after passing through many lives, cities, and times, covering the east and west coasts of the United States and almost one decade of the 20th century.

George Ohsawa visited Paris via the Siberian Railway without any financial support and then published his first book, *Unique Principle*, in French (Vrin Company, Paris) in 1931 at the age of 38. More than forty years have passed since it was first printed in France. We are very happy and proud that we are able to publish this in English at last. We are sure that this is a great book for people who wish to study Eastern philosophy and its application in the various fields of science. However, the most important contribution of this work to modern society is in the fact that it will lead people to a better and deeper understanding of the principle on which Eastern religion, morals, character, living customs, and science are based. And this understanding, in turn, will help people lead happier and healthier lives.

On this Thanksgiving Day of 1971, I am so grateful to everyone who has helped to make this publication possible, especially to Lou, Armand, Fred, and Joyce for their translating, editing, and typing; and to Ken Burns for his work revising the *Tannishyo*. Also, many thanks to Marvin Mattelson for the cover design and I have no way to name the many people who remain anonymous who donated their time and work to realize the dream of having this publication printed.

– Herman Aihara
1973

Contents

Introduction

To offer to the Western World a key to the philosophy and science of the Far-East, one which at the same time opens the mysterious door of the so-called "primitive mentality," is a daring gesture for an Oriental to make. This key is the "universal law," the "unique principle" of ancient Chinese philosophy and science more than fifty centuries old.

Today, the Orient is so taken with the importance of the dazzling civilization, philosophy, and science of the West that few Orientals take any serious interest in their own ancient philosophy and science. Everyone recognizes the *I-Ching (Book of Changes)* and the *Ni-Ching (Canon of Houang-ti)* as the surest sources for them but no one studies these overly famous prehistoric books with a philosophic spirit and modern scientific approach. A few Japanese doctors study the *Canon* very superficially, and this only in their capacity as "doctors," but disregard the *I-Ching*; a few Japanese philosophers read the *I-Ching*, but never the *Canon* except as "philosophers." However, the ancient philosophy is actually grounded in science, and the ancient medicine depends entirely and solely on the philosophy. It is impossible to understand one or the other without having deeply examined the ancient fundamental ideas, which are expressed in the theory of the two activities Yin and Yang.

I shall call this theory *In'yology*. In'yology is the most positive philosophy of the Far-East. It embraces all sciences. I believe it best enables the Westerner to understand Buddhism and, thereafter, all the most profound philosophy of the Far-East where all the practical sciences of life—medicine, biology, economics, and sociology, for example—are found in one extraordinary and harmonious synthesis.

"Did the philosophy of the Far-East ever exist, or does it exist now?" I am asked.

"Yes and no."

If the goal of modern Western philosophy, such as the philosophy of Kant, is "to know oneself," the Orientals had and still have something analogous to it. At least that much can be said. But the philosophy of the Far-East goes beyond this point. It is indeed a deepened, delicate, and most complete study of the theory of knowledge similar to that of Kant; furthermore, it is practical to grasp and easy to follow by everyone. It goes beyond the confines of simply knowing oneself. It is a practical culture, ethical, scientific, and esthetic at the same time.

In the Orient, it is forbidden to analyze and reconstruct fundamental knowledge in any manner. Truth, beauty, and good are each only one interpretation of the unique, all-embracing law. They are "several equal to one." They must never be considered separately, not even in imagination. One cannot have a perfect conception of universal law by synthesizing it bit by bit from various pieces. The "river" could not be reconstructed even if one were to gather all the drops of water that apparently formed it. In the Orient, instead of analyzing, one must widen the synthesis, ever more endlessly unifying all knowledge and, above all, one must practice it in daily life.

Lao-tse has said, "Without practice, no virtues."

Ancient Chinese philosophy, as well as that of the entire Far-East embraces both a theory of knowledge and its application to practical existence.

"Has the science of the Far-East ever existed, or does it exist now?" I am asked.

"Yes and no."

Western science has for its goal the perfect knowledge of the chronological sequence of phenomena, in order to profit from them. It is active and positive. Oriental science, on the contrary, is negative and passive. A perfect understanding of the law of order is its starting point, not its goal. That is to say, it does not carry on any research—it has no need of it—but it strives to live and utilize the perfect knowledge confirmed to it by philosophy, its sovereign to whom it is faithful and obedient.

According to Augustus Comte, human understanding developed from theology, went to metaphysics, and reached positivism. In the Orient, it appears to me, it has been the reverse. Knowledge developed from positive science and reached divinity via metaphysics. It finally achieved the perfect understanding of the highest unifying principle.

From its beginning, science in the Orient has been perfectly governed by philosophy. The wise man, the great philosopher, was the one who arrived at a perfect understanding of the unifying principle that governs the causality of all the phenomena of the universe. Ancient Oriental science explains the system of the universe and all the phenomena that occur in it by the law of *In'yology*, somewhat as modern physics is explained by the atomic theory. The theory of Lavoisier in chemistry has its equivalent in the law "Musyonin," which says exactly the same thing about matter.

But the use of science was strictly by philosophy. One might say that science is the scaffold of the great philosophical structure; it no longer has a reason for being when the latter is erected.

But even if theoretically we do away completely with these differences between Western and Oriental philosophy, on the one hand, and between modern and ancient science on the other, there still remains another very great one. It is the fact that philosophy and science are but one in the Orient. Philosophy is the sole fruit of science—it is the awaited ruler who, once born, will govern all of science forever. The synthesizing scientific research of the ancient peoples led to the perfect understanding that permitted them to grasp the intimate nature of all phenomena. It is absolute knowledge in the face of which neither time nor space exists.

It is the sublime unique law that explains past and future just as it does the present, the invisible as it does the visible, the imponderable as the ponderable, that which cannot be heard as well as that which can, the mineral world as well as the organic world. Were it only a simplistic system produced by an overly naive imagination, we should at least respect its theory and study it seriously to cut from it the few bits that might be interesting to us from the historical point of view.

In'yology, that is to say, the unification of science and philosophy, was invented by the ancient Chinese emperors. The activities Yin and Yang, which are the basic units presented to us by this philosophy, constitute all the phenomena, assimilate one another, and almost represent $\gamma \lambda \eta$ of the physiologist DuBois-Reymond. But *In'yology* offers, beyond this, that which produces $\gamma \lambda \eta$. We shall examine it later.

All that I have said until the present concerns ancient China, because I will deal solely with the formation of the spirit of the Far-East through philosophy and science, from its prehistoric origin until the 5th century before Christ; that is, until the period when Confucius, Lao-tse, and Shakyamuni began to enlighten the world. There is nothing of further interest following this period from our particular point of view because philosophy and science had already been perfected prior to this time; the subsequent march of history only brings us discussions of minute, useless details due to the superficial or erroneous comprehension of the fundamental principle. It is the slow march of decadence in China, India, and Japan.

There have been no additions or rebirths of *In'yology*. Today, only fortune tellers and magicians pay any attention to it. It has been abandoned and misunderstood by men of science. Its true significance, so practical at its origin, has been lost. It has been clouded over by enormous symbolic difficulties. The only reason it has not totally been lost is thanks to its amazing simplicity and to the record of Confucius' study of it via the *I-Ching* during the last twenty years of his life.

The great Buddhism, Mahayana, has disappeared in China and India. *In'yology* has disappeared everywhere. Such is the present condition of the philosophy of the Far-East. Can it grow again or is this the final spiritual fall of the Oriental people?

In order to grasp the unifying principle of Chinese science and philosophy, one must bear in mind that the mentality of the Orient is in every way the antipode of the Western mentality.

At first glance, its philosophy appears negative as opposed to positive. In reality, it is above objectivity and subjectivity.

Neither its science, its religion, nor its philosophy require or demand any propaganda whatever; on the contrary, they insist on secretiveness. "Hide the truth," says the wise man.

The truly traditional education does not have exterior and material knowledge as an aim. It only wishes to teach us our own smallness and ignorance of ourselves and strives to develop to the highest level the practice of the "instinct-intuition" (see "Theory of Knowledge," Part 2).

The logic of daily life is the opposite of the West. The least example can prove it. An address is given in the following order: the country, the city, the street, the house number, the name of the recipient.

Syllogism differs likewise.

And, in daily life, the greatest and smallest extremes are always ruled out; one states the conclusion only. If one should say to any uneducated worker in Tokyo:

> "You are mortal because . . . ."
> "Berabo-me!" (You are an idiot!)

...he will interrupt you before you are through speaking. Reasoning is unbearable and much too heavy for Orientals due to the traditional training of the intuition. Such is the cause for the relative lack of skill of the Japanese in international diplomacy. Ordinary reasoning is more or less scorned by tradition and, even more so, the analytical scientific reasoning. The conclusion alone must be expressed in as precise and as limited a choice of words as possible. In the course of my Western studies during these last two years, the greatest difficulty I have found has been acquiring the habit of Western word expression. At all times, under all circumstances, I used to state the conclusion only. This appeared at first incomprehensible, then annoying, bothersome, and strange to my French professor.

Our conversation without any apparent reason seems mysterious to Westerners. One example:

> Shakyamuni Buddha one day showed a flower to the dis-
> ciples gathered near him, saying, "Today I am yielding
> to you the entire secret of our philosophy—this is it."
> No one seemed to understand him. A single disciple
> smiled, looking at him.
> "You have understood me. I give you permission to
> teach in my place," said the Buddha. Even he did not
> want to create any detailed explanation.

Simplification is the order. For example, in Buddhism the entire
philosophy, which was dealt with in innumerable books, has been
systematized into the 600 volumes of *Maha Prajna Paramita Hridaya Sutra* (see Appendix), which in turn have been condensed into
a mantra (master-words) of 17 or 18 syllables, and finally into one
syllable: *Aum* or *Om*.

The spirit of the philosophy best shows itself in the simplest
form; words hide its true nature.

The secret of Chinese science and philosophy is also condensed
into two words: Yin and Yang, the theory of the polarized monism
that I will explain in Part 2.

According to tradition, never must the secret of the philosophy
and science of the Far-East be translated into an analytical form.
However, I have been the first one to violate this unspoken rule. The
unifying principle itself has never been clearly presented. From antiquity to the present day, no book, no document expresses the twelve
theorems of the unique law; I have purposely formulated them for
the benefit of the West. This is an untenable procedure according to
tradition. Therefore, I shall not show them to my Oriental students.

Not only have I explained the unique law in a manner more or
less modern, but I have developed it into a theory of being and a
theory of knowledge; furthermore, I have been led against my will
to offer several applications in the specialized sciences. These are
enormous sins. Everything is explained to an inexcusable degree.

Nevertheless, all this may still appear vague to Westerners. Certain scientists are already asking me for more detailed explanations, charts, a complete classification of foods, of produce, of vegetables and animals according to *In'yology*. We do possess such complete charts: the medical encyclopedia that Li-Che Tohen published in 1578 after devoting 26 years to its study. But a classification is not very practical because of its essentially relative and changing nature. This will be understood well enough later.

I would say that one ought to strive to grasp the unifying principle of the philosophy and science of the Far-East without dissecting it through analysis. One must understand fully its pliability to learn how to apply it to all of modern science. In order to reach this peak of understanding, I believe, there is only one road: constant and ever-deepening reflection. This too-detailed exposé must be abandoned after it has been well assimilated in order to meditate on the substance of it at every moment, in order to read it in daily occurrences. (Note-taking is actually scorned in Oriental teaching of all *In'yological* or traditional science or philosophy.)

The theory of polarized monism of *In'yology* has an organic mechanism invisible to mechanical researchers. It is like the "flying arrow," out of reach of those who want to possess it through analysis; once one has grasped it, it no longer is the "flying arrow." But if one considers it as an abstract movement, the *arrow* no longer exists.

Chronology

I confess that I am not profoundly interested in the chronological question because the Oriental mind has no bent for this kind of order, which requires extreme precision. Orientals can only present all the possible material about their tradition without any exaggerated explanation.

The traditional chronology that almost all the modern Oriental specialists accept is the following: Fou-Hi, 2900 B.C.; Sin-Wong, 2780 B.C.; Houang-Ti, 2640 B.C.; Iu (Ou) 2200 B.C.; Tcheou-Kong, 1100 B.C.; Confucius, 552-479 B.C.; Shakyamuni, 564-484 B.C.

But certain scholars do not follow these dates. Some of them take the period of Fou-Hi back as far as 8,000 B.C. Others deny entirely the historical truth of all these great personalities. My teacher, M. Nishibata, for instance, does not accept the existence of Houang-Ti. He believes that the *Canon of the Emperor Houang-Ti* was written somewhere in the 2nd and 1st centuries B.C. by an unknown writer. As yet, I cannot publish my own chronology, nor am I acquainted with the chronology of Chinese development established by Western scholars, having busied myself with the study of natural and physical sciences since my arrival in France. I have not read the French sinologists; I have only thumbed through Chinese science as presented by Prof. A. Rey in Book VI of *Science Orientale dans L'Antiquite* and have found it precise.

My chronological order is not precision-bound and has two foundations. The first is biological; the second is a general biological philology, which should not only define the etymology of the Chinese, and especially Japanese, language, but must be a fundamental contribution to general philology. Part one of my study is completed—I have discovered biological particulars of a remarkable nature:

1. All the great men, all the emperors, and all the ancient philosophers were incapable of perceiving light rays below 4900 or perhaps 4400 Angstroms. Therefore, they were all blind to blue, indigo, and violet.
2. They had a great many more teeth than modern man.
3. Their breathing and their pulse were much less intense, etc.

I have deduced from these particulars and from the disappearance of them in the race something new from the chronological point of view.

I shall wait several years to publish my conclusions.

Furthermore, for several years I have had a rather childish notion that the prehistoric Chinese, at least under the reign of the "three augusts," inhabited land quite other than China as it is known today.

The solar eclipses in the period Hia observed by the Chinese at the observatory of Fond must have been produced, according to the calculations of Goubil, on the darkest nights at this location (see the *Science Orientale* of Prof. A. Rey). The witnesses that described them, therefore, must have lived in a country other than modern China. This fact permits us to suppose that the observatory was situated at 70 or 80 degrees longitude west. It is well known that any people who emigrate take along with them the names of their native sites.

Further, I want to obtain permission to consult and to copy, if possible, the *Canon of the Emperor Houang-Ti* in the oldest edition kept as a national treasure at Ninnaji Temple in Kyoto. If one could discover the old books that the expedition of the Emperor Tsin-Chi-Houang brought to Japan before the great fire of the year 213 B.C., the actual chronology would be greatly clarified.

The Chinese Science and Philosophy

The Origin

To reveal the unique spirit of the Oriental people in its origin and development from the purely philosophic, psychological, and scientific point of view is the goal of this treatise.

Let us go back several thousand years....

One of the primitive nomadic peoples that has been roaming over the whole continent of Asia settled at an unknown period on the plateau of central China. The plateau is vast, naked, and devoid of humanity for the most part, an ocean of hills and dales melting into the sky at the distant horizon. Sprinklings of hamlets are seen here and there.

The sun is setting far off on the high plains.

A man emerges from one of the huts in the central village. His name is Fou-Hi. He is the leader of these people. His figure is massive, solid, gigantic—like a statue chiseled with a few simple, vigorous strokes of utter precision. His hair reaches to his shoulders. His long beard is black, his nose straight and high, his eyes large, brilliant, and penetrating.

He strides forward with long elastic steps, solid and vigorous as those of a young man. He reaches the terrace, which reveals the view of the entire plateau unto the most removed fields. The wind has ceased over the corn field from which the moon, full and yellow, rises.

The philosopher-leader contemplates the sky, where the stars have already appeared. This has been his custom of several years. Night progresses....

His age is already beyond 80. In his youth, he had been the most active warrior, the one worker who knew no fatigue. He had struggled against innumerable difficulties—war with outside enemies, internal strife, famines, great forests, etc.—and he had succeeded in overcoming them by guiding his people. His fine memory and intelligence enabled him to supervise the agriculture, cattle raising, and other primitive industries of his country. He was familiar with all the needs of their lives. All obeyed him spontaneously with respect and even with pleasure. Later on, when he became the official leader, everyone was satisfied under his rule. Peace and prosperity flourished; it was a golden age. He was able to devote his time to the contemplation of, and reflection on, all the phenomena of the earth and the universe.

He established the science of astronomy. He synthesized all hereditary knowledge accumulated from generation to generation. He had a rather large group of collaborators and assistants occupied with philosophical and scientific research under his direction.

First, they sought the cause of each phenomenon, which later directed their research into the ultimate cause of all things. They sought it at all levels for years and years. They analyzed everything, criticized and examined minutely all the results obtained. Their methods were necessarily crude in the realm of experimentation, but they verified their results most carefully, and in the end, deduced a fundamental cause. They then grouped the various causes thus obtained and pursued their induction to the end. By means of intuition and Oriental meditation, they sought the essential cause and made efforts to achieve universal synthesis.

The alternating recurrence of light and darkness was first of all considered. The one was a benefactor of humanity, the other its enemy. This regular alternation (coming and going—origin of all vibration), which makes us work, which allows us to rest, which makes the leaves shoot in the springtime and makes them drop in the fall, was indeed the fundamental phenomenon. The same coming and going, the same opposition, was discovered in all of nature. When day ends, the night does not delay its coming. Before night departs, the day is already prepared. Therefore, day is the beginning of the night. Therefore, nothing is ever complete, finished; all things are evolving, dependent, and connected. Birth is already the seed of death.

The physical exterior of our existence and the spiritual interior of our life are nothing but one more example of this universal oscillation of opposites. One climbs the mountains and there discovers the factors that distinguish the plain: ocean and land, animals and vegetables, organic and inorganic, hot and cold, fire and water, etc.

The philosopher-leader characterized these innumerable opposites two by two into two separate categories. In the first were found the following relative properties: light, solidity, elasticity, resistance, compression, heat, weight. In the second: darkness, softness, flexibility, fragility, expansion, cold temperature. . . . Always guided by pure intuition, he was soon brought to interpret these properties by their activities, which were far less numerous; that is to say, constriction, weight, centripetal force, on the one hand; dilation, force of ascension, centrifugality, on the other hand. He named the first of these activities *Yang* and the second one *Yin*.

He did not cease his contemplation.

It was on one evening of this period that we watched him leave his hut and reach the terrace. He was continuing his profound contemplation. Toward midnight, two or three shadows, as roughly hewn and statuesque as himself, carrying enormous bundles of logs, appeared on the same terrace. They were his collaborator-assistants, come to make a fire for their master. The flames were brought to life. The fire was kindled it and illumined the master and his faithful disciples.

First, the master made a worshipful greeting to the fire. Then they all sat themselves around it. They did not speak but continued their contemplation while gazing into the flames. Night deepened. The bright moonlight illumined the whole meeting place with a bluish mist. The philosopher-leader was looking very intently into the fire, as if he were reading something in it. All of a sudden, he motioned with his head and spoke: "Yang attracts Yin, Yin attracts Yang."

This was the law long sought by him. He explained slowly and at length in measured tones.

"Fire is evidently Yang, and it has and must have the following characteristics: constriction, gravity, and centripetal force. In effect, it possesses them all. But air, the atmosphere, being Yin as our intuition indeed senses due to its coolness, its dilation, and its eccentric movement is completely in opposition to fire, Yang. These contrary forces cannot but attract each other. The fire, being less powerful and smaller in size than the air, which is infinitely more vast, is attracted to the power above. That is the reason why the flames rise. One activity always attracts the opposite activity, just as day and night follow each other attracted by one another, just as a woman attracts a man. The fire travels up into the air and continues until all its heat finally transforms itself into cold. Yang produces Yin; Yin produces Yang."

By turning his intuition and his deepened reflection to the universal vibration to the perpetual oscillation of the two activities, he understood necessarily that everything is in motion, eternally, without ceasing, and that this motion itself varies in time in an exact and regular manner. Nothing is at rest in the universe.

He penetrated deeply into the darkness of contemplation. Finally, he found that this obscurity was full of substance, the nature of which was comparable to nothing in the world of light, but that it possessed a particular activity that gave forth to motion, and that this activity itself must be pronounced by two opposed activities that attract one another as is shown by all the phenomena of the world. These former are the ultimate cause of the latter.

He went far deeper in his meditation but explained himself only up to this point. He designated what he sensed at the heart of his metaphysical work by the word *Taikyoku*, which I shall translate not literally, but philosophically by the expression "essential nature," or the "ether-universe before polarization." It designates that which constitutes the entire universe and consequently all the beings in it. For ourselves, *Taikyoku* can be understood only in its two manifestations according to the activities Yin and Yang in their multiple composites. In other words, essential nature manifests itself through Yin-Yang activities.... One can understand the ether-universe before polarization only by intuition; no word can convey its meaning.

The wise one judged it futile for men to penetrate further into their studies because the principle of the two activities suffices to explain the world on all its levels. Therefore, he did not invent any sign to interpret *Taikyoku*, but he symbolized the first Yang activity, the positive point of departure of our world, by a quadrangular stick in order to give his disciples a concrete example and to simplify his teaching.

"*Taikyoku* produces one," said he.

Although "one" symbolizes the first Yang activity, it must not be considered as the arithmetical number 1. Numbers, which are perhaps the first scientific invention of mankind, had an extraordinarily deep significance in antiquity, especially in China. The number 7, for instance, is considered as a Yang number, and its positive multiples have particular meanings. In many realms, in physiology for one, this number is very important. The age of 7 distinguishes boys from girls. Their physiological differences begin to be accentuated and, from that time on, they are kept strictly apart until marriage. This separation prepares for a more enduring communion. Year by year, it increases the positively-charged Yang activity among the boys and the negatively-charged Yin activity among the girls. At the age of 14 (7 x 2), menstruation occurs; it is the third physiological period. With each following period, there appears a more or less striking physiological phenomenon; in particular, the change of the pulses of an individual in relation to his age demonstrates this clearly. Menstruation ceases at the age of 49 (7 x 7).

I will not take the time to explain at this point why the number 7 is so vital, nor why it is the father-number of 5, 7, 12. (5, 7, and their sum, 12, are the foundation of poetry as in *Haiku*, *Waka*, or *Alexandrine*; but also of music: the Chinese scale of 5 basic sounds and the Western scale of 7 tones. The 7-color spectrum is also within this category.)

"One produces two," continues the sage. Here we understand

that "two" is the two activities, Yin and Yang; this is the polarization of the ether-universe. These two give rise to all living and inert beings. If we translate "three" as all possible beings, we have then: "One produces two; two produces three; three is manifested as all possible beings."

This last sentence was most cherished by Lao-tse.

In this statement, one sees set forth the theory of polarized monism and the theory of the evolution of the universe and all creation. The Yin-Yang theory is not ordinary dualism because there is no being nor any phenomenon purely Yin or purely Yang; all are extremely varied manifestations of the possible combinations of these two activities. The theory of evolution, which follows from this understanding, is quite different from that of Darwin. If there is a relation between biological beings at the level of the cells, or at the realm of the function of their organs, this proves that the fundamental life force is one and the same; the principle of one life, in effect, is single, unique: it is the oscillations of the activities Yin and Yang in infinitely varied proportions.

If life is a manifestation of the two fundamental and universal activities, it can produce itself at all levels, be it in the depths of the sea or on a high plateau—of necessity assuming different forms according to the milieu and the time—because any being is its transformed environment, no being existing independently of its surroundings. The living organic creature, as well as inorganic phenomenon, can have as many origins as, and even more than, the species because the manifold conditions of environment are infinite in reality.

The philosopher-leader symbolized Yin and Yang with three quadrangular sticks of the same size. In the center of each one, he whittled an indentation equal to the width of the stick but 1/3 its depth. One side of the stick is a solid plane; it is the symbol *Yang*: compact, solid, contracted. The same piece of wood turned over on its other face shows the indentation that signifies *Yin*: separated, dilated, receptive, hollow. Yang and Yin are but the two faces of the one stick (*Taikyoku*). When Yang appears, Yin, below, awaits its turn at any moment. The polarization and the antagonism between Yin and Yang (hence the rotation and fundamental vibration of all systems) are marvelously translated by this squared piece of wood; I shall name it the *Stick of Logos*.

Two Sticks of Logos arranged in a cross, Yang over Yin, form a figure that is neither Yang nor Yin on any side. It is the communion between Yang and Yin; it is the secret symbol of Buddhism and of diverse sects and schools of traditional teachings; it is the talisman of various superstitious faiths, the symbol of the gracious harmony between man and woman, the supreme dynamic balance between the activities Yang and Yin. The swastika of the Buddhist religion is a variation of this sign. This same philosophical cross is the basis of all sacred symbols, such as octants and two juxtaposed octants softened or modified into flower petals or into geometric designs.

In order to enlighten his people, the wise man interpreted all the fundamental phenomena of the universe with these three Sticks of Logos: astronomy, meteorology, the physics of water, the chemistry of fire, life, death, all social and individual occurrences, agricultural science, ethics. Let us imagine his method:

First he takes up one stick and places it flat in the Yang position: ——

"This is the symbol for the earth. Let us examine it: at this state it is Yang, that is to say, activity and strength dominate it entirely. Look—everything is lively, everything is busy, all is vigorous."

Having said this, he places another stick parallel to the first one in the Yang position: ==, and he continues, "The second one symbolizes the sun. It is the sun of summer; it is full with Yang activity. It sends us more light and more heat.

"In these positions, the two sticks represent the Yang sky and the Yang earth; this symbol is called the *Great Yang*. The sun be praised! It is strength; it is the light that protects us, which gives us all the products of the field, of the streams, and of the mountains.

"The sun is truly the source of Yang; it is the Yang of Yang. Thus, these two sticks show us the world in the time of summer when the sun, Yang of Yang, sends us more heat, when the earth overflows with Yang activity, rich with life everywhere. All of this teaches us what we, the sons of the Earth and the Sky, must do: labor. It is our expression of thankfulness towards the sky and the earth. Let us work in order always to be on good terms with these powers. For soon ... see, see carefully ... on the reverse of the *Great Yang*, the *Great Yin* (symbol of winter – –) is prepared; all is inert; all is frozen and arrested; death reigns here. Therefore, let us work now. Summer is the proper time for activity. He who labors is happy. It is our time of gratitude to the sky, our appreciation to the earth. Never let us forget that wintertime is already waiting on the other side of the world. Young men, this is your time. Apply yourselves as industriously as ever; you shall then have some abundant harvests. Old men! Work along with the young ones—guide them. You shall earn a satisfying rest in the following season."

The philosopher turns over the upper stick. Another symbol is obtained: $==$. It describes the diminishing heat of the sun. The autumnal equinox has passed ... one feels the coolness in the air. Fall ... the waning of life; death soon approaches.

He names this symbol *Small Yin*. Time travels on without ceasing.... The leader turns over the other Yang; this is winter itself. It is the time for rest. One must be very cautious. It is the period of $==$, the *Great Yin*. The earth is clothed in melancholy. All appears immobilized. But time continues endlessly.... Here is the spring equinox now. The upper stick turns over $==$. Spring is here. The sun's warmth increases day by day. On the mountains, the snow is thawing, the rivers rise, the grasses sprout, the rains come fine and gentle. It is the *Small Yin* that heralds coming summer.

Thus, the philosopher-leader preached the universal cycle with four permutations of the two squared sticks. He then added another stick. With these three pieces of wood, he found eight permutations.

He continued his teaching. His orders, intermingled with prophecies, were taken solemnly and mystically by his people who all obeyed him without question. If he declared war against barbarians, his army was victorious; if he ordered close conservation of the crops, famine was understood to be near; if he had the dam repaired, the floods were on their way.

He included in his teaching not only natural phenomena, but those pertaining to social, family, and individual life—always having recourse to the same principle, the change and pulsation of the two activities. At this point, I feel it important to give a brief sketch of the philosophy of the three Sticks of Logos.

The three sacred sticks represent the entire universe. The first one (the one that is placed uppermost) represents the sky, that is to say, the astronomical and meteorological conditions, or the climate in a general sense.

The third one (in the lowest position) represents the earth, the geographic, economic situation, etc. The second one (the one that is between the other two) represents all that the earth and the sky produce: creatures and phenomena, universal and terrestrial. The first stick is called the Sky. The second is Humanity, representing all beings. The third is the Earth.

The first permutation is obtained by placing the three Yang sticks ☰. This permutation is called *Ken*, where the Sky, Humanity, and Earth are all Yang. It symbolizes plenitude, good balance, the magnificent evolution of the great nature of the universe. If we consider politics, for example, *Ken* stands for "peace." In dealing with the realm of agriculture, it signifies successful tending to the necessary tasks and predicts an abundant harvest because the weather (the Sky) is clear and normal, man (Humanity) works with all his strength, and the Earth is represented by well-tilled, well-watered fields.

An equally good balance is indicated by the inverse of *Ken,* which is called *Kon* ☷. If one contrasts *Ken* with *Kon* in cosmological terms, *Ken* stands for the sky and *Kon* for the earth. In a sexual sense, they are male and female. In ancient traditional biology, they are father and mother, land and sea. In the study of orientation, *Ken* is northwest in China, for example; *Kon* is the opposite direction. This applies only in central China where the southeast is open lowland that runs into the *sea* (dilated, humid, soft). *Ken* (Yang) produces vapor (Yin) from the earth. Vapor goes up by its Yin activity—centrifugal tendency of ascension—and is directed by the constrictive, centripetal power of mountains (Yang) that concentrate the vapor in the air. The concentrated vapor falls to earth. The cycle closes. The same cycle revolves between man and woman; man absorbs all that is Yin and condenses it, purifies it, in order to extract its essence, the male sperm, an accumulation of Yin activity that is the origin of the feminine sex (see the later discussion of parthenogenesis). Woman absorbs everything that may be Yang in her environment, condenses it, purifies it, in order to form the ovule (Yang), that is to say the masculine germ (I refer you to Part 3 on Yin-Yang biology). The animal species feeds on the vegetal realm and decomposes itself into minerals at a certain time; the vegetal kingdom feeds itself on minerals and grows, thanks to its specific expanding power. The male fecundates, and the female brings up. Man builds, and woman undoes; they are antagonists, enemies as it would appear, but dependent on, and indispensable, to each other.

☰ is considered a Yang symbol because the minority is here represented by Yang; it is always the minority that rules on all levels of life. This symbol, for example, signifies a sociological and political state of blind souls that are governed by a wise head. Peace reigns here. The Sky and the Earth are Yin, melancholy, dull and relaxed; but the beings, Humanity, are seething with activity (Yang), its people are well-disciplined, it is a well-tilled land. If such a sign were attributed to a human being, it would describe a well-developed person—socially and outwardly gentle because he is surrounded and sheathed by soft Yin elements but extremely strong at the core.

Among natural elements, the symbol would apply to water—for instance, water that obeys all, that adapts itself to all sorts of molds, that is quiet and modest but that has the power to bear extraordinary pressure; water that carves a path through massive rock in order to regain its goal, the ocean.

"Water is humility itself; it falls at everyone's feet; it listens to everyone; it lowers itself for all; it penetrates everything; and it crosses all obstacles. Ultimately, nothing can prevent it from doing what it has to; consequently, it understands all, it feeds all, it unifies all. Kings, administrators must possess the qualities that are demonstrated to us by the very nature of water," states the wise man.

and subjectivity. *Taikyoku* appears as it is.

Let us take an example: the arrow in motion.

An arrow flies from A to B by crossing space. If one were to consider it subjectively, and one were to follow it with a categorical knowledge of space and time, there is a series of positions A, A', A", etc. In order to fill the spaces between A, A', A", one multiplies the intermediary positions to the infinite. However, one gets nowhere in solving it. Some strongly declare that the question has no solution; others still insist that it is a discontinuity, etc....

All speak the truth, as they have different points of view. Some are objectivists, some subjectivists, while some are intermediaries. If one sees it from *Taikyoku*, the ether-universe, there is nothing at all—neither movement nor discontinuity. If one bases his reasoning on time and space, fiction of our consciousness, one arrives at "continuity" via subjectivism and "discontinuity" via objectivism. To clarify these ideas, let us use as proof a cinematographic film of the arrow from point A to point B, an imaginary distance of 10 meters, with a speed of 100 meters per second. Let us imagine a highly efficient projector capable of containing 2400 pictures per second (10 times more than the G. V. of Debrie, 150 times more rapid than an ordinary projector). This proof, image by image, gives a superb backing to those who prefer the theory of continuity. However, if this film is projected at the rate of one still per second on an ordinary screen at the correct distance, perhaps 10 meters, with a powerful lens—let us say 50 millimeters—the separation between one still and another is clearly observed. There is the foundation of the theory of discontinuity. But if one takes away the screen, if one projects it into infinite space in the imagination, there is neither continuity, discontinuity, nor movement. In the same way, it is impossible for us to know the absolute movement of all the stars.

Some say that neither good, beauty, nor truth have a concrete existence. Others claim the contrary. But neither the first proposition nor the second have any meaning because neither one group nor the other know in reality what existence is. Thus, from time to time, one comes across certain realities created by imagination and human contrivance. (Stereo-chemistry, for example is the convention which holds that such or such molecule is long or short: CH_3 - CH_2 - CH_2 - CH_2 - CH_2 - CH_2 - CH_2 - CH_2 - CH_2 - CH_2 - CH_2 - CH_2 - CH_2 - CH_2 - CH_2 - CH_2 - CH_2 - CH_2 - COOH, or HF.)

In order to see the image of *Taikyoku,* one must close one's physical eyes and open the eyes of the soul. (The ancient Chinese invented two different verbs corresponding to the verb "to see"— to distinguish the physiological faculty of seeing from the spiritual faculty of seeing—and two different words for these two eyes, the physical eyes and the spiritual ones.)

One needs the latter for the search of being, the searcher of the true universe being somewhat like a photographer. The closer the eyes come to the object, the more the field is contracted; at the closest possible distance and with the most powerful lens, they pick up an incoherent image. The farther back the viewer goes, the more he enlarges his field. At an infinite distance, if that were possible, he would get a perfect image of the object in its totality within its entire environment, the true universe, from which he could then examine, with the appropriate instrument, all the details that he had taken close up. One must not stubbornly insist on objectivity or subjectivity. The invention of new methods of viewing things analytically or microscopically only gives a relative gain, one of size on a sliding scale. One does not progress into the understanding of the nature of an object, which is the cause of its properties.

In the Yin-Yang theory of being, the origin of life is altogether resolved. Ideas such as panspermy, actualism, heterogenesis, *Generatio spontanea seu acuinova*, abiogenesis, etc., are not necessary. Did some plants, for whose reproduction certain butterflies are necessary, exist before the creation of the butterflies or not? Likewise, does the egg come before or after the hen? These questions are only capable of being solved from an understanding of *Taikyoku,* like the problem of the arrow, or movement, or matter.

The Theory of Knowledge

Is the true nature of psychological phenomena beyond our grasp? Such a question has no place in the philosophy of the Far-East. Spirit is considered as one phase of the essence of nature; the other is called matter.

One considers that all beings, all phenomena, including our entire existence, exist within the true being, within the true universe of *Taikyoku*. Psychological phenomena produce themselves within the womb of true nature as well as all physical phenomena, all beings. "Phenomena are the language of true nature (*shiki soku ze ku*)." Spiritual phenomena are nothing but the movement—the force, if you wish—of the spirals that we had found in the depths of the ocean, which was the ether-universe of *Taikyoku*, bubbles or froth, insignificant yet infinite, which appear and disappear in the water of the aquarium of true being. They are, therefore, nothing but beings dependent on their environment, true being; they are a consequence, a state of balance of neighboring reactions, and of the being that is at the same time the universe and the beings that it produces.

If one wishes to learn only the law of ephemeral being or actions that govern these bubbles, without wishing to know the universal law that governs the ephemeral beings and at the same time the true nature, one will never achieve his aim because he himself is one of these bubbles.

It was in the philosophy of the Far-East, and particularly in Buddhism, that one studied the theory of knowledge with the greatest of care. I shall leave aside the theory of the five elements and the theory of evolution in twelve stages as quite superfluous to us at this point.

We shall enter into the spirit of the general theory of knowledge of the Far-East. Here, we are, looking down on the entire world, the world of our existence that extends itself in the universe of true being. We understand that our world, our existence, our life, everything is nothing but a spark produced by the contact of the two activities Yin and Yang at the heart of *Taikyoku*. We represent *Taikyoku* by a certain point: our physical existence begins with the polarization of

Taikyoku. It ends with a perfect saturation, a neutralization that is represented by inertia, which is followed by a total decomposition, ruled by new activities, finally becoming a new communion of opposite activities. But our spiritual expression is maintained forever; this is *Taikyoku* itself, root of our life, soul, or native country of all beings. *Taikyoku* and ourselves, beings, are but one. We are *Taikyoku*. This is the mentality of faith. When we shall grasp this—as soon as we shall not understand but sense *Taikyoku* throughout our entire existence—we shall be freed from the prison doubly encircled by time and space. From then on, we shall see the past and the future as well as the present under our very eyes, at once, in their microscopic details and in their totality. Just as the focus of our physical eyes is instantaneous, in the same way, our spiritual eyes—marvelous windows viewing onto *Taikyoku*—recognize instantly what is on one far side, the past, and on the other far side, the future; as well as what is found close by, the present. The faculty of focusing on the past is memory; when applied to the future, it is intelligence; and for the present, it is knowledge. Memory, knowledge, and intelligence are only three focusing positions of one instrument.

I wish to call this instrument *intuition*; it possesses the faculty of regulating itself automatically; it represents *instinct*. (This self-adjusting mechanism is more or less defective in the majority of persons due to lack of perfect health.)

I call *recognition* the exact focus at each position.

It goes without saying that by means of this miraculous lens, with self-focusing power on all levels, I am representing the *Perfect Intuition-Instinct*, that is to say, Intuition beyond the reach of various influences and equipped with a perfect instinct.

With us, the lens and the regulating mechanism are not independent, as they are in a camera.

The totality that possesses this exactness, this perfect function of automatic adjustment of the instinct, is the only instrument at our disposal to contemplate *Taikyoku*, the true universe. It is a miniature *Taikyoku*; it is a microcosm and, at the same time, a part of the macrocosm, *Taikyoku*. Provisionally, I shall call this masterpiece *Perfect*

Consciousness or *Taikyoku Consciousness*. (What is difficult to understand is that this microcosm and this macrocosm are really one because they are part of one another.)

The *Primary Sensation* is, therefore, in Oriental philosophy the elementary recognition at the cellular level; the developed and combined sensation is neural recognition.

Spirit is considered as a tendency and a stage of development of the system *consciousness-understanding*. Sensations, emotions, feelings are the elementary recognition, as we have stated previously. The majority of persons cannot deny them because they are elementary; that is to say, they are physical, material or, in other words, they are at the root of our physical existence, of our birth, at the center of our spiral, which is sensitive and whose function—rotation—is troubled by a foreign obstacle.

Consciousness, such as we have defined it, is the antipode of *knowledge*. Within *consciousness*, we can deny the *self* without feeling pain because *consciousness* is the summit tree, the furthest periphery, the one most removed from the root center of our spiral. In this area, the foreign obstacle does not upset the movement very much; its periphery melts in the infinite water, ether-universe, *Taikyoku*. There is no obstruction of continuity between *consciousness* and *Taikyoku*.

Wants and *desire* are formed by distillations of various sensations that have been classified into certain determined tendencies.

The *Idea*, the *thought*, are considered as the synthesis of *knowledge*. Empiricism, or the objective theory, strives to seize the external tangible characteristics of phenomena without taking into account their intimate nature, which is the source of all their properties. It translates them quantitatively by certain conventions (mathematics) while always using subjective logical categories, such as time and space. The science of Yin-Yang is not interested in this objectivity that inevitably leads to abstractions. It is neither objective nor subjective. It melts into *Taikyoku* by the deepest contemplation, while freeing itself of the *self* which is the inventor of objectivity and subjectivity. These two approaches to understanding are grounded in the existence of man, in his personal capacity. *Taikyoku* is beyond both. The ancient Chinese or Hindu philosophy does not allow us to justify our existence because we are man, a bit of ephemeral form. It is, at the same time, the theory of *consciousness*, the true universe.

We shall explain several rather common problems by observing from now on the terminology that we have heretofore established.

Does the accomplished fact exist in space?

This question is badly put. If we examine what space signifies in the theory of consciousness of the Far-East, we shall find that it is a human convention and has no meaning in the true universe. The same applies to action, the fact. The question melts away like a rainbow.

Are scientific forecasting and scientific explanations possible?

Modern science is a research into causality on all levels. But through analysis, we can find only the preceding cause or a multiple of preceding causes and never the ultimate one. One has already modestly declared "Ignoramus" as well as "Ignorabimus." But, aside from the ultimate cause, is prediction possible? Certainly. I do believe it. A science that works tirelessly and modestly should be able to arrive at scientific prediction after numerous and lengthy re-searches. But the so-called scientific prediction does not go beyond the level of probability because it limits itself to *knowledge*, which has already been defined. The idea of causality itself is subjective.

Are forecasting and explanations possible according to In'yology?

Consciousness (always following our own terminology), being without solution of continuity, foresees everything as well as *Taikyoku*. To reach this state is the sole goal of the entire philosophy of the Far-East. Forecasting, according to the *In'yological* technique, is also perhaps only a probability based on *knowledge* but also on *consciousness*. The scientific probability based on causality could be compared to a juxtaposition of infinitesimal numerous photographs of a large object taken at a distance of 0.1 meters; whereas, the

In'yological forecast is like a single photograph taken at a distance of perhaps 1000 meters, a suitable one to project the whole object within its environment.

What is Good, Beauty, Truth?

These are reflections of the Unique Law of *Taikyoku* seen by the *consciousness*, either in the realm of morality, esthetics, or in the domain of science.

The Good must be freed from its more or less persistent subjectivity; the True must always mistrust its objectivity; only the Beautiful is perfect. He whose *consciousness* functions perfectly finds beauty everywhere. He is always happy. He is man who puts everything into poetry or a sincere and grateful person who has faith.

The Self and Free Will

The *self* as an object of meditation is the physical *self*—the human being—a phenomenon or a state of dynamic equilibrium at a given moment in the course of oscillations and vicissitudes, which vary infinitely between the forces Yin and Yang at the center of the ether-universe, *Taikyoku*; consequently, such a *self* has no freedom whatever.

The *Self* that meditates (on the *self*) is the spiritual *Self*, which is neither passing phenomenon nor a particular state of dynamic tension, which is the ether-universe, *Taikyoku*, or *Shunyata* itself; consequently, its liberty is perfect and absolute.

At a certain stage of innocence, this meditating *Self* is worshipped and is sometimes called *God*, in respect, or *Soul*, in friendly rapport. That it inhabits the smaller *self* (the physical one), that death is its exit and life its entrance, is held in naivete.

Without knowing either small *self* or greater *Self*—that is to say, neither all the beings nor the true Being—all discussions on free will are useless.

Once upon a time, one imagined a donkey deprived of free will, and one asked oneself, "If this donkey is positioned at equal distances from two equally large and savory haystacks, would this donkey perish of starvation due to lack of free will?" It would appear that the animal would perish, but, luckily, the instinct-intuition of the donkey replaced the so-called free will of the scientist. I believe that the latter must have his focal apparatus blocked by knowledge in relation to the objective, which is the instinct-intuition. In other terminology, the perfect functioning of the instinct-intuition is the consciousness representing *Taikyoku, Shunyata*—therefore, perfectly free.

He who possesses it is the man who knows the *Tao* of Lao-tse. He is the "perfect man" of Confucius, a Buddha. This is the sole personality that the entire philosophy of the Far-East strives to achieve.

He, who through his existence, is in touch with the true universe, *Shunyata*, belongs to no religion or to any sect. It is always the disciples and the listeners who create religions and particular sects because they lose the true essence of the teaching.

The universe and existence are the visible world of *knowledge*. The one and the other are created solely through physical perception (of time, space, and gravitation).

The invisible world—the metaphysical or spiritual world—is the image of the uncertainty of existence, of the anxiety of the inhabitants of the visible world.

Universe or existence, plus the invisible or metaphysical world, are but a geometric point in *Taikyoku, Shunyata*, where neither time, space, nor gravitation exist.

Subjectivity leans on the individual knowledge of the inhabitants of the visible world. Objectivity leans on the general knowledge of the function of the units CGS (centimeters, grams, seconds). The difference between subjective and objective is not qualitative. The philosophy of *Taikyoku, Shunyata*, is above both of them; a mentality that is either subjective or objective is absolutely incapable of interpreting the philosophy of the Far-East.

The consciousness of *Shunyata* or *Taikyoku* itself is called Perfect Consciousness. Understanding, God, instinct, intuition, large self, *Daiva*, or *Nirvana* are nothing but a partial expression of Perfect Consciousness. What distinguishes one of these expressions from

COSMOLOGY OF THE FAR EAST

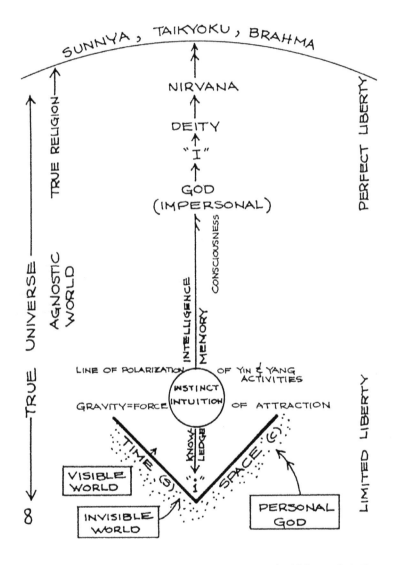

Schematic representation of consciousness *around which gravitate the* visible world of self and the invisible world of the self.

ation these notions with the system of the Far-East. Man inhabits at the same time the visible world by his body and *Taikyoku*, the world of Perfect Consciousness, by his soul. The forgetting or neglecting of the soul is the true source of all physical and moral ills of humanity.

All so-called religions, which require rites, observances, penance, prayers, which predicate a Paradise, a Hell, a personal God, etc., or which do not deny their usefulness, belong to the visible world and are considered pseudo-religions in the philosophy of the Far-East. A "True Religion" is one that bypasses them to save perfectly humanity from every kind of ill and suffering.

Monotheism, polytheism are terminologies useful only in the visible world of knowledge and absolutely useless in *Taikyoku*.

When one enters deeper into the small *self*, the frame of time and space narrows, restricting one's freedom, and if one struggles against this limitation, with the help of the only powerful weapon one has, which is called analysis, one ends up with the abstract zero, or even beyond zero, toward the negative infinite. But if, on the contrary, one directs oneself toward *Taikyoku*, *Shunyata*, by means of contemplation, after having passed the frontiers of the two activities of Yin and Yang, one arrives upon *consciousness* and melts into *Taikyoku*, *Shunyata*.

Instinct, Apriorism, Posteriorism

The instinct has two activities, two extremities: one is intuition, the other is consciousness. The perfect and automatic function of our apparatus, the instinct-intuition, is Consciousness itself.

I shall leave aside all the discussions of the definitions of apriorism and posteriorism, and I shall start with the conclusion that Oriental philosophy offers on this same question.

It admits of no posterior development of knowledge. The development, the deepening, the enriching of knowledge are an illusion provoked by the growth of the apparatus. It is simply a difference of scale.

This is the illusion one meets when one goes in the direction of the small insignificant *self*, struggling against the tightening hold of time and space and ending up in abstraction. Toward the end of one's life, one feels that it is useless to have sought so persistently to know it. (Many end their lives without feeling even this.) Modern physiology, for example, shows us great strides, but it bravely asserts "ignoramus" and "ignorabimus" about all fundamental questions, such as the exact composition of a protozoan or the mechanism of the cellular function.

The posterior knowledge, in any event, does not make us progress. A newborn baby or an organ acts like it should without having any "posterior" knowledge—that is to say, instinctively, perfectly.

Practice precedes reasoning; that is, the instinct is predominant in our system of understanding. Instinct is perfect on all levels of the natural world and forever, from birth to death. Knowledge itself does not exist without instinct. Instinct does not develop nor does it grow weaker as one's life goes on. But one pampers oneself by looking for verification of one's instrument, the instinct-intuition, and one lingers on its threshold immobilizing it to the point of no return by drowning it in details. (The instinct and the intuition are but one.)

Chinese or Hindu philosophy does not discuss posteriorism or apriorism. By means of contemplation, it removes our illusory existence where there is no screen that holds time in ordinate, and space in *abcissa*, and on which the beings are projected as defined creatures.

The difference between a child and an adult, or between a bushman and a Newton, is thus cleared up. This does not at all mean that I admire instinct and that I scorn knowledge. One must not exaggerate. If anything, I rather admire modern science—monument to the glory of knowledge—which I have recently learned. Some souls, more or less insignificant, worship instinct and intuition and like to bury them in a secret box of mysticism, or the coffin of knowledge.

The Dream
The astronomer only has to replace "T" (time) in the lunar equation with a certain positive or negative number to know the occur-

rence of a solar eclipse at any given period of the past or the future. If physiological knowledge could arrive at such a sure road, we could establish a cerebral equation that would apply to the functioning of a brain that is capable of sleep without dreams. But as soon as the dream would make its appearance, the equation would lose its validity. "No scientific knowledge will ever allow us to see the mechanism that connects our human brain to the dream," says Du Bois-Reymond.

According to the ancient philosophy of the Far-East, dreaming is a disturbance of the "consciousness." (During the night, the Yin hours, consciousness withdraws into *Taikyoku* or *Shunyata*.) There is no dream in perfect sleep; our entire consciousness is in perfect communion with its point of origin, the heart of the universal mother, *Taikyoku*, from where, resting, it finds renewal of strength. But if there is any kind of physiological imbalance, the imperfect consciousness, that is to say "Knowledge," dominates our body in sleep. Knowledge is always imperfect; therefore, our thoughts, our dreams, are incoherent.

Mong-tsu has said, "Hiziri (the man who fully knows *Shunyata Taikyoku*) has no dreams at all when he sleeps." Dreaming is a symptom of illness states the medicine of the Far-East, violating the Law of Man, which is the physiological law of the Universe.

"If Hiziri should dream, it would be a true dream," says a Chinese philosopher. A true dream is pre-vision. When one is in perfect harmony with the Unique Law in the practice of living, one does, occasionally, dream the events of the future. It is logical and natural to foresee what is to come when the consciousness is in perfect communication with *Taikyoku*, where neither time nor space exist. The history of the great men of the East has given us several such examples.

The Word
Words or speech develop in parallel with human knowledge and inversely with our consciousness. The cause and origin of words, of language, is knowledge.

Finality

One who has understood the simplicity, the regularity, and the exactness of the Unique Principle understands causality perfectly. Yin produces Yang because Yin is not Yang. Heat finally turns to cold because heat is the opposite pole of cold. The queen bee lays exclusively male eggs; it is the small island (environment) that creates the dwarf. (See Chinese Science, Part 3.)

Reality

We have already seen that the past is one distant horizon and the future another. For myself, Japan is the past when I am in Paris. For you, it might be in the future if you have never been to Japan. For my friends in Tokyo, it is the present. My young children do not distinguish it at all from either future or past; for them, the entire world is one unity where there is no time or space; they are not yet very far from the world of *Taikyoku*.

One considers the present as a reality and the future or past as a dream. But Japan can be a reality—that is to say, the present or a dream—or the future or the past, according to the point of view of the observer. Likewise, for some people, the life of Christ is in the present. It is a far away island in the infinite ocean of time, just as Japan is in the ocean of space. In reality, be it the existence of Jesus Christ or the existence of Japan, it is only a geometric point within *Taikyoku*, which one distinguishes either by the chronological point of view or by the geographical one.

Let us suppose that you are the victim of a storm, trapped for more than one month on a small sailboat without a rudder, awaiting almost certain death. At such a time, the world toward which you were sailing, where your children are awaiting you, is nothing but a dream. But as soon as you are rescued by a large ship whose arrival at a major seaport is already determined and expected, that world recaptures its concreteness; the dream transforms itself at once into reality, and you are no longer uncertain about it. Perhaps, however, this very ship, a glorious testimonial to modern technical achievement, will sink two minutes following your rescue, as happened to the Titanic. To tell the truth, this entire universe is only a Titanic that is crossing the ocean of *Taikyoku*. It is fragile and ephemeral, although it is believed solid and enduring as it is called "reality." One despises the eternal dream. In some ways, people are like the fisherman who prefers the catch of a small fish today to that of a larger one tomorrow, without having determined whether that very small fish might be the cause of his death, so blinded is he by physical, immediate pleasures.

You are a builder of ships. After long hours, you have now finished the plan for a new ocean liner. At that moment, the ship is a reality for you; it will appear as a dream sometime after it has been constructed. However, it is absolutely impossible for you to find a solution of continuity because you had your very first idea about its design.

The true poets, the true composers, do not have objective awareness of themselves while they are working. Their work is a dream for their friends. The accomplished work of art is a dream for them, but a reality for their friends.

One cannot find discontinuity between dream and reality. The emissions caused by sensual nightmares, frequent among young people, are another example that do not allow us to separate dreams from reality. One is quite conscious of the physical sensation.

We must, therefore, declare that our consciousness creates our reality. Our reality depends on our mental functions. The same is valid for all psychological functions as are dealt with through hypnosis, psychotherapy, dream analysis, etc.

Westerners consider reality that which occurs within the frame of time and space; the peoples of the Far-East consider it just a dream.

For the latter, time and space, fiction of consciousness or of modern science that strives to interpret all phenomena through abstract mathematical notions, are a fiction and a dream.

In brief, reality is held to be fragile and passing, and the dream is divided into two categories that are both 100 percent accurate in their own respect: (1) The dream strictly speaking—that which takes place in our disturbed consciousness during sleep; and (2) the dream of our consciousness, which sees equally well the past as the future, be it in sleep or in a waking state.

The present is a fleeting point, insignificant when viewing the entire past and future. Strictly speaking, it is only a function of time and space. Within it, happiness, freedom, joy are equally insignificant and illusory. No one can grasp perfect and eternal happiness in such an ephemeral world. The Great Joy, undeniable and indestructible, is only to be found in the world of *Taikyoku*, *Shunyata*, where freedom and strength are perfect. Orientals call it *true reality*. This is the world of which *Maha Prajna Paramita Hridaya Sutra* gives us a glimpse and toward which the *Words of Shinran* steer us through the ocean of small reality, a pitiful state, where storms and good weather alternately torture and cajole us until we reach the far shores of the landing port of our native country—The Great Joy.

Modern science is erected on the reality of the present. Time, space, gravitation, all unexplained knowledge are considered occult and mystical in the philosophy and the science of the Far-East that, freed from these illusory notions, has its foundations in *Taikyoku*.

Chinese Science

Chemistry

We have examined how Fou-Hi made every effort to resolve the problems of the ultimate origin of beings as well as of the purpose of creation, and how he succeeded in establishing philosophy. His means were: First, experience, and then, contemplate. If I call "philosophy" the principle discovered after his long studies, I must label "science" the means by which he could arrive at this principle.

Instead of tracing the history of the science of Fou-Hi from its start to its perfection, as we have summarily done for philosophy by the Sticks of Logos, we shall attempt to interpret it partially, and just as roughly, in a fundamental modern science, such as chemistry, and in one branch of practical application representing modern science, such as biology; then we shall review as examples of the application of Oriental science native and traditional Chinese medicine. We will thus be able to understand and judge the ancient science, its usefulness and vitality.

In order to translate ancient science into the terms of modern science, one must have a rather deep knowledge of both. Unfortunately, I have not had the time to make a profound study of modern Western science; therefore, I shall examine only some representative examples, while waiting for the Western people themselves to take interest in the subject.

I believe that chemistry was the one science most favored by Fou-Hi and the ancient emperors. I might go so far as to say it is the basis of all ancient Chinese science. What distinguishes it from modern chemistry is that it sought after the cause of the properties of the elements, their very nature. We shall examine the law of Fou-Hi

SPECTROSCOPIC CLASSIFICATION OF ELEMENTS

RED	ORANGE	YELLOW	GREEN	BLUE	VIOLET
↓ 6500	↓ 6000	↓ 5750	↓ 4820		↓ 4290

H

He

Li
C

Na
5896

Ne
Mg
Cl

B
N
O
A P
Si

Be
F
P
S
A

Sc
Cr
Ni

Ti

V Ca

K
Mn

4044

Fe
Co

Cu
Zn
Ge

Ga

As

Se
Br

Kr Rb Sr

Y

Zr
Nb Mo

Pd

Ag

Cd In

Rh Ru

X Sb

Te   I

Cs
Ba

Ce

La

Sm

Nd Pr

Em
Tb Eu

In Ta
Hg Pt Au
Th Te Ra Bi

Dy Ho Er Tu
W Os Pb

YANG ACTIVITY ⟶
(WEIGHT)
CENTREPETALITY ⟵
CONSTRICTOR)
HOT

YIN ACTIVITY
(FORCE OF
ACSENSION
CENTRIFUGALITY
DILATION)
COLD

by interpreting it in terms of modern chemistry. It still proves applicable, or at least logically admissible. We must admire the good sense of the ancient philosopher-researcher to research into causes, and if we inquire into his experimental technique, if we imagine the simplicity, the naiveté, the crudeness of his means, we must be overwhelmed by his wisdom.

Can the law of Fou-Hi still operate in modern chemistry as it does in guiding the entire philosophy of the Far-East under the particular form called the "Oriental spirit?" I must confess that I so believe it, and I shall prove it briefly by an examination of the affinity between elements, which I consider a fundamental question.

We must not, according to *In'yology*, attach ourselves to the various properties of elements, but seek that which produces them, without setting up any hypothesis.

The radiation produced by elements under identical conditions seems to me to characterize their nature better than all the other properties singled out by Western science.

Spectroscopic examination will allow us to give a measure of the index of the Yin and Yang activities. We already know that long waves (red) and short waves (blue) have opposite tendencies; the first ones have more heat and are excitable; the second ones are cooler and calmer. Consequently, the first ones are Yang, and the second ones are Yin. Thus, we can consider the very spectrum as a reflection of the essence of nature. The ultra-violet or infrared spectrum are other reflections of it. The law of photo-magnetic resonance of Helmholtz is implied in the 10th proposition of the Unique Law.

Aside from the elements themselves, one must classify all factors and agents according to their nature. We can then explain all chemical reactions, including affinity. (I shall leave aside the cases where the secondary spectrum of absorption plays a principal part in the place of the vanished principal elements.)

Spectroscopic Classification
 The adjoining chart is divided into six columns:
  lst, starting from the left, comprises all wave lengths above

6500 Angstroms
2nd, radiations from 6499 to 6000 Angstroms
3rd, radiations from 5999 to 5750 Angstroms
4th, radiations from 5749 to 4820 Angstroms
5th, radiations from 4819 to 4289 Angstroms
6th, radiations below 4289 Angstroms

The symbol of each element is placed under the corresponding column of wave lengths within the major spectrum of absorption. The choice of the latter has been made from the *Atlas Typischen Spectren* by Dr. J. M. Eder and Prof. E. Valenta, with the table composed by M. Kaysner. For certain elements such as F, CI, and I, due to lack of documentation, I have been compelled to position them according to their affinities, the relative actions. An imaginary line divides the whole diagram into two sections running through the center of green.

Its place is determined before hand between the two neighboring complementary colors. The elements placed to its left are characterized by the Yang activity; those to its right are characterized by the Yin activity. These activities manifest themselves in variable degrees, but it can be said in a general way that for two given elements, whatever their position might be in relation to the imaginary central line, the one farther to the left will be characterized by Yang, the other by Yin in their relation to one another. The elements are classified according to their nature Yin or Yang. Their attractions and repulsions explain chemical reactions, for even the external determinants, the physical agents, the balancing factors, are also classified Yin or Yang, and this is always relatively so for, as will be seen, nothing is absolutely Yin or Yang.

We can sum up, from the chemical point of view, what we have just said in several simple propositions that govern both the affinities and the reactions of elements.

Relativity of the Activities of Elements
1. Every element has its own special action, Yin or Yang. In the

same manner, all compounds are specifically Yin or Yang in infinitely variable and relative degrees.

2. Yin and Yang activities are antagonistic.

3. Yin and Yang activities attract each other. If a substance is stable (which is never so, strictly speaking), it is due to a neutralization of its own tendency by an opposite one.

4. Every chemical element and every physical element represent a combination of activities. One cannot be considered separately from the other.

5. The greater the distance between the elements within one category, the greater the force of attraction between them, the attraction between elements comprising them.

6. The closer their proximity, the more the elements repel each other.

7. Elements characterized by the same activity—close neighbors to each other—do not combine. To achieve their combination, one must put into effect a Yin activity if they are Yang, and a Yang activity if they are Yin. Examples:

    a. C does not combine with H. To achieve this, one must have some Yin factor such as ultra-violet rays. Thus: 2H (Yang) + ultra-violet rays (Yin) + 2C (Yang) = C_2H_2 (Yang)

    b. N does not combine with 0. To achieve this, one must have some Yang factor such as heat. Thus: N (Yin) + Heat (Yang) + 20 (Yin) = NO_2(Yang).

    c. $(CO_2 + H_20)$ x Radiation of Light 200 micro-angstroms (Yin) » CHOH (Bail, Baker, 1921)

    d. (CO_2H_2O) x Mg » Formaldehyde (Fenton)

    e. $CuO + H_2 = H_2O + Cu$ shows that their power of attraction or of repulsion varies with the distance that separates the elements in the chart. The distance between O and Cu is smaller than the distance between O and H.

8. A powerful source of Yin or Yang activity can change the Yin or Yang characteristic of any system, for example, heat (Yang) and ultra-violet rays (Yin).

9. Na is representative of the Yang category; K representative of the Yin category.

10. The various states of dynamic balance must be represented by equations that take into consideration not only all comprising elements but also all physical and chemical agents.

11. By use of the spectroscopic classification, it is possible to grasp the origin of particular sciences that are founded on one major and clearly characterized element. For example, C and organic chemistry; H and ionic chemistry; Na-K and Oriental bio-medicinal chemistry, etc.

12. The denser elements behave as a Yang activity in relation to less dense elements, which behave as Yin activity.

13. The elements located in the middle section of the chart participate in two activities in more or less stable balance. (Halogens, catalysts, precious metals, etc., all possessing the so-called "mystical" properties.)

Yin-Yang Explanation of Several Chemical Phenomena

1. Br (Yin) doesn't combine with Au (Yin), nor with Pt (Yin). (Example of proposition 6 above)

2. $2H_2$ (Yang) and O_2 (Yin) combine easily, both being essentially different natures. (Proposition 5 above)

3. H (Yang) is replaced by Li (Yang) in the cathode, for the latter is stronger in Yang activity.

4. $3Fe + 4H_2O = Fe_3O_4 + 4H_2$. Why does H separate in this reaction and not O? Because: [Fe (Yin) + Heat (Yang)] + [O (Yin) + Heat (Yang)] = [Heat (Yang)] x [Fe (Yin) + O (Yin)]. But H being Yang doesn't combine with Heat (Yang) and goes into the air (Yin).

5. *Antagonism Between Calcium and Potassium*: Ca and K differ but little, according to our spectroscopic classification. However, some scientists will point out their antagonism in physiology and in medicine. This occurs because methods of preparation, of solution, have transformed the nature of Ca, which has become Yang in relation to K.

6. *Phosphorous—White and Red*: The chemical equation repre-

senting the transformation of white phosphorous into red phosphorous is P=P.

However, the differences are strongly noticeable: the smell, the degree of fusion, the individual form, etc., and above all the toxicity; 0.1 gram of one is sufficient dosage to kill a man, whereas the other cannot be absorbed by the human organism and is eliminated intact. According to *In'yology*, white phosphorous is a Yin element to a considerable degree, as are its neighboring elements—oxygen, nitrogen, fluorine, sulfur, etc.

However, in the case of red phosphorous, this Yin activity is neutralized by the heat (Yang) to a certain extent. One therefore has the equation: P (Yin) x Heat (Yang) = P (Yang) or, more specifically, P (Yin) x Heat 230° (Yang) = P (Yang).

Heat can be replaced by light. Chinese chemistry takes into serious consideration that which is found within the parenthesis, that which is invisible but implied, whereas modern chemistry predominately centers on that which is tangible.

Biology

Now we will begin to read the Unique Law in the biological realm. According to *In'yology*, all living beings, just as all forms of nature, must submit to the general laws of the physical, material world. Ancient science does not allow any hypothesis here any more than it does in chemistry. Heredity, evolution, struggle for survival, etc., are here reduced to their ultimate cause: the two activities Yin and Yang.

Seaweeds and Their Topographical Distribution

There is a species of black seaweed called *hiziki*, and others resembling it, that live at great depths in the ocean. These are unknown in Europe but are a favorite in Japan and of great therapeutic use. (In the Orient are many occurrences not admitted to, unknown to modern Western science.

In the case of *hiziki*, one may say that it adapts itself to its environment, adjusting to the darkness. However, such an adaptability is not a voluntary adaptation of the seaweed. The correct way to say this is that light, lacking in long wave lengths [activity (Yang) and water (Yin) absorbing 80 percent of red wave lengths at a depth of 10 meters and 100 percent at a depth of 20 meters] cannot allow any kind of existence but an extremely Yang one in such Yin surroundings. Stated otherwise, living beings are created and nourished by their environment.

In principle, each species of nature must be the particular creation of a particular environment. That which differentiates and characterizes this environment is nothing but the manifestation of the complex action of the two activities Yin and Yang. The same species can very well appear in any location and at its antipode at the same time, if the conditions are identical. It cannot be said all species have been derived from the same origin at a given time at a given place.

If there are signs of an overall relation between the species, it is because the substance (the universe and beings in it) is the same for all, as well as the productive force (all the physical factors) and the laboratory (the earth).

Determination of Sex and Parthenogenesis

Let us take some one hundred eggs. We can very easily divide them into Yin and Yang categories. It goes without saying that those of the first group are elongated in comparison with the rounded ones of the second group. The first ones are male and the latter are female because Yin produces Yang and Yang produces Yin. It is not at all a question of probability; probability only exists for man's mind. By and by, chemistry will prove that the first ones, male, are greater to the second ones in all Yin elements (represented by K) and that the latter are greater in all Yang elements (represented by Na). In the same way, the spermatozoid is long and the ovule is round. If the vitality of the ovule is stronger than that of the sperm, their communion will produce the male sex, and vice-versa according to the law. This is the deciding factor of minority: ☲ (Yang) and ☵ (Yin). (In the first trigram the middle line ⎯ is the deciding factor; in the second trigram the middle line – – is the deciding factor.)

The woman (Yin) produces the ovule (Yang), and the man (Yang) produces the sperm (Yin).

Climatic, geographic conditions, and various (not easily measured) factors play a most important role. Thus, all factors being equal, there are more girls than boys born in lands that border the sea, where the Yang activity, as represented by Na, predominates; and more boys than girls in the mountains. (This is why the Mormon religion, originating near the great Salt Lake, must allow polygamy.) In this respect, islands are the opposite of mountains. Legendary sirens did not dwell in the mountains. *Nyogo-ga-Shima*, the female-dominated part of Japan, where women work instead of men, is a small island. The dwarfs, contracted beings because of Yang activity, inhabit islands. Note that a Yin continent can be transformed into a Yang country by special conditions, that is, if the food contains many Yang animal products, if there are great deposits of salt, if there are hot springs, etc.

In the same fashion, an island changes into a more or less Yin country due to humidity, to cold winds from the ocean, etc. Temperature as well as degree of light play a capital role. If the inhabitants of an island with a hot climate—therefore an island dominated by Yang—feed themselves largely on vegetables, potatoes, yams, which are incomparably high in K (Yin), they grow quite large, that is to say, dilated by the Yinnizing influences. The opposite is true for the inhabitants of an island of colder climate, as the English people, for example, who consume Yang foods and are of moderate size.

Today, these are the insurmountable difficulties that prevent accurate statistics of a nation's population from giving testimony for the Unique Law. At the time of Li-Ki in China, there were yearly counts of the population and the statistics (dating back at least to 500 B.C.) of a country where the nutrition was a correct reflection of the environmental conditions, giving quick proof of this law.

The female bee, or queen, lays eggs, some of which receive the spermazoid. The non-fertilized egg (ovules, Yang) always give rise to males (Yang) because they were deprived of the Yin influence from the sperm and were absolutely dominated by the Yang of the ovule. Yin, the queen bee, produces Yang (males). She mates only once in a lifetime. All her fertilized eggs produce females. In this case, the sex is determined at the very instant of fecundation. The virgin eggs charged with Yang activity always give birth to males.

The determination of the sex thus depends to a large degree on the chemical elements, although it is not the sole factor. Again, one must take into account the physical agents. Heat, cold, dryness, humidity, atmospheric electricity, light, darkness, magnetism, atmospheric pressure, any unusual stimulus, etc. all play a very important role and more particularly among the lower, simpler levels of creation. One simple excitation, whatever it may be, can be a Yang or Yin factor according to the case. One must understand here that reproduction, sexuality are nothing but an oscillation, a vibration of Yin-Yang activities. The phenomena of parthenogenesis demonstrates it. Certain animals, as a result of parthenogenesis, produce exclusively one sex, Yin or Yang, for one season (also Yin or Yang); and because of another factor, produce or can produce both sexes at another time (the green fly, for example).

If the number of chromosomes serves to determine the future sex, it is because that number itself is determined by Yin or Yang activities.

Morphology and Physiology to the Vegetal Realm

All physiological functions (the shape, the size, the color, the sound, tropism) are equally ruled by the Unique Law among plants as among animals.

An undersized plant, quite pale, can form stalks ten times longer in darkness (Yin, dilation) than one exposed to the light (Yang, contraction). The sexuality and the formation of the leaves, of stalks, etc. can be grouped under the morphological function; sexuality is nothing but the formation of the sexual organs, which is what modern plant physiology accepts and demonstrates by numerous examples.

According to Nobbe, Erdman, and Schroder, buckwheat does not form starch (Yang) in the absence of K (Yin, expansion). It is very hungry for K. The Japanese peasants have known this for a long time. This characteristic must be considered seriously in therapeutic application.

K is an integral part of all plant tissue. It is a very important constituent, whereas the amount of Na always varies more or less. Certain plants, such as the tobacco plant and the potato, absorb Na with great difficulty. (M. Maquenne.) K is the Yin representative that is indispensable to plant life—fundamentally Yin—whereas Na— Yang representative—is less necessary. (The case is quite different among animals.)

Certain plants lose their color and turn yellow because they are subjected to an excess of lime or of magnesium carbonate (M. Maze, 1913.)

There is, therefore, an excess of Yang elements, whence the yellow coloring (Yang). In the same way, the brown leaves of fall have a Na content much higher than that of spring leaves. Beets (red) and carrots (orange) are also rich in Na. (The mountain carrot of the renowned Korean *ginseng* is one of the major ingredients that enters into the preparation of various revitalizing aphrodisiacs of the Far-East. The use of an iron container is strictly forbidden in the preparation of *ginseng* because it kills its root; iron is strongly Yin and *ginseng* is Yang. What delicate sensitivity among these philosopher-doctors! No Japanese doctor can find an explanation for this decree. What crude sensibility among the moderns!)

Plant Respiration

The activity of breathing among flowers and of germinating grains is much more intense than that of other parts in other stages of plant development. Flowers and grains are the parts of the plant richest in Na (Yang representative) and require more oxygen (Yin). Outside of the period of flowering and of germination, the intensity of plant oxygen requirements is always lower than that of the assimilation of carbonic gas (CO_2). This latter activity is sometimes 10, 15, 20 times more intense than the former. The taking in of oxygen and the breathing out of carbonic gas in humans is a function of Yang activity because oxygen is explicitly Yin (therefore characteristic of animals, Yang). The assimilation of chlorophyll is a contrary function, Yin, because CO_2 is explicitly Yang (it is a product of combustion, Yang). Plants breathe out Yin oxygen because they are essentially Yin.

In the study of Chinese biology, one holds that plant respiration is the inverse of animal respiration.

Respiration must be understood to designate the general function of absorption of various types of gas, not exclusively oxygen.

Fruits and a Dry Climate

The maturation of fruits is accelerated and perfected in a dry year. (M. Maquenne: *Precis de physiologie vegetable.*) In a general sense, fruits are very rich in K (Yin representative) and consequently thrive in heat and dryness (both Yang) at the time of their ripening, which is nothing but a communion of the two opposite activities. Yang produces Yin. There is a Japanese saying: "A dry season, the perfect ripening of the melon!"

Animal Respiration

Animal respiration is the opposite of plant respiration. The first class has great need of oxygen (Yin), much more than the second class. Tables dealing with the respiratory quotients of various fish by M. M. Bruntriol, Kanamaru, Paryo and other authors clearly prove it. The carp or the eel can live in water singularly deficient in oxygen but rich in CO_2 in the wintertime, showing that they are both quite Yin creatures (under the combination of the Yin dilating, centrifugal, quieter activity). This characteristic of the carp was put to use in ancient Chinese medicine. No modern prescription is as efficient as the "stew from the living carp" to heal pneumonia or croup. (Note that winter is the Yin season, and that the carp, also Yin, has less need of oxygen [Yin] during this season). On the contrary, very Yang fish are of small size—all other factors being equal—and are much more active and quick-moving, all Yang characteristics. The herring is one example.

Animal Heat
Body heat is necessarily related to respiration, and the latter is a function of Na/K, all other factors being equal. If animal heat is controlled by the surface temperature of an animal, the latter depends solely on the Na (constrictive)/K (dilating) ratio, all other factors being equal.

In a general way, the intensity of the breathing, the heart beat, the pulse, and the carotid pressure are much greater among those whose diet is rich in Yang elements. The blood is "cold" when the K content is relatively high, representing all the Yin, cold elements.

Cellular Polarization
This insoluble enigma of modern physiology is implied in the 12th proposition of the Unique Law. Yin (-) rises to the surface and attracts Yang (+).

Na and K Among Plants
One can find a great number of examples of Yin-Yang activities in the thesis by M. D. Perietzeanu (K and Na in Plants, 1926). From the *In'yological* point of view, one can draw the following conclusions, which are an explicit confirmation of the Unique Law in all phenomena of vegetal life.

1. The coexistence of Na and K, representing the two fundamental activities of life, is universal among plants.

2. The ratio K/Na is always higher than the one characterizing animals, generally speaking, because plants are relatively more Yin than animals, as *In'yological* plant morphology teaches us.

3. Within the same species, plants express their particular K dilating and Na constricting ratio in each case, according to their individual morphology.

4. Na and K are opposite elements that complement one another in the manifestation of plant life; both are indispensable, just as in animal life.

5. The content of K and Na among plants depends on the species, the origin, the growing area, and time, all other factors being equal.

(Example within one species: wheat, winter and summer).

6. Examples from differing species: corn develops a larger root in a solution rich in Na due to its centripetal Yang activity, contrary to the reaction of another plant for which an equal amount of Na would not be sufficient to satisfy its own well-established necessity. (The nature of tropism becomes clear).

7. In an environment where K has been completely replaced by Na, the vegetation finally perishes for lack of an essential dilating factor.

8. In an environment where Na has been completely replaced by K, vegetation develops perfectly due to the expanding force provided by K which allows it to attract Yang, of which the minimum quantity is sufficient for Yin realms of life (Yang of carbonic gas, of luminous radiation, of the air).

9. The chronology of the flowering period is also a function of the Na/K ratio, according to the species, the origin, etc.

Man and all animals perish like plants under the influence of Na in excess. A certain amount of Na can kill a child very easily. (The same with other neighboring elements spectroscopically classified such as As, Hg, Ra, etc.) But a certain quantity of Na and K is defined according to the Unique Law. All physiological and biological phenomena are functions of this particular proportion: tropism, morphology, cell metabolism, etc.

I stop here with my endless quoting of examples to end with the words of the French scholar Laplace:

"Infinitely varied in its effort, nature is only simple in its causes, and its economy consists of producing a great number of phenomena often very complicated by means of a small number of general laws."

The Medicine of the Far-East

Preliminary Observations

Although there are numerous European books that translate with great care the Chinese ordinances, these merely bring out very Occidental characteristics of Oriental medicine, which are certainly the least interesting ones because the medicine of the Far-East has three reasons for being:

1. The first and highest is to guarantee the physical and, above all, the moral health of humanity, subject only to the Unique Law and liberated from all restricting and boring rules.
2. To cure any illness to come.
3. To cure any present illness. This is the third, which is considered the lowest and easiest goal.

One might be inclined to smile or be surprised to see that the last, therapeutic medicine, so difficult for modern science to accomplish, is considered the last and easiest goal to achieve. Traditional medicine, incomparably difficult to learn and much altered by superstitions, is actually only known to a few *Hiziri* who have voluntarily removed themselves from society. Strangers who would study the art would not know how to recognize these men among the host of so-called traditional doctors who are profoundly ignorant and self-seeking. The following lines written by a foreign doctor who lived in China more than ten years will demonstrate how the lack of the necessary philosophical, chemical, and biological understanding of the Unique Law can totally eclipse so-called traditional practice.

"A Chinaman will spend ten cents for a prescription, obtained to put the genie of a cholera epidemic at rest, for instance, but will paste a counterfeit receipt for five francs on his door, hoping that the evil spirit, so deceived, will not dare to cross the threshold of such a generous man to put this man's family on his list. This childish trick gives him great security. These deceptive tactics are also employed in the realm of the official hygenic precautionary rulings. During the great epidemic of the plague in Canton in 1895, the authorities, wildly alarmed by the spreading disaster, found nothing better to do than to change the dates of the official calendar and proclaim the first of January to be three months behind its actual time. The reasoning was that the genie of the epidemic would notice when he reached Canton that he had arrived three months too early and would not fail to leave the city and its inhabitants in peace."

The absolute ridiculousness of these measures is evident if one would stop at these observations, but the careful observer might notice that there is mention of a complete change of diet and way of life. No doubt the Chinese only saw in this a religious observation of purification, of a necessary vow under the circumstances, but the basis for it was purely biological. The very physician who reported these facts as well as the Chinese themselves were totally oblivious to it.

Koempfer, much the superior observer to this modern doctor, reports some very interesting items in Japanese medicine of the 18th century. Those affected with smallpox were wrapped in a red sheet, and if the patients were the children of the emperor, the clothing of the servants attending them was red also. If one knows the K content in the dye traditionally used to achieve this color— known as the "precious red of Beni" because it was an extract from the plant of the same name—one understands the efficiency of its vibrations, which are Yin, to cure such a Yang disease. With the same understanding, the Japanese employed the "red of Beni" for the lips to relieve a fever from menstruation (Yang symptom) and also to alleviate chapped lips (Yang). A bit of silk dyed with this particular color relieves eyes suffering from trachoma.

Little children are traditionally dressed in red, which bathes them in the radiation of K; unfortunately, today the "red of Beni" is replaced by aniline dye, which is incomparably cheaper and extremely Yang. Therefore, women suffer from cracked lips and children from skin inflammations. The mortality of the latter in Japan is among the highest in the world.

The Only Law of Chinese Medicine

The only law of Chinese medicine is explained in four words, *Shin do fu ji*, which means man is the result of his environment. In other words, to maintain natural and perfect health, man must feed himself on the products that nature offers him in his environment in the very same proportions as they are naturally produced. This refers, of course, to the natural, that is to say traditional, products that might be found within a 50-kilometer radius from his dwelling place.

It is neither vegetarianism nor carnivorism. Modern carnivorism, which ignores historical biological chemistry, has more against it than for it in physiological considerations. However, animal food can be tolerated by the human body if man remains within the limits of the law of environment. Thus, the inhabitants of a very cold region (most Yin according to our terminology) can and do have a diet that is almost entirely animal (consequently Yang). Whereas, the inhabitants of tropical countries (extremely Yang) are almost entirely fruitarians and vegetarians (Yin diet).

Vegetarianism, ignorant of this law of the environment, is as dangerous as carnivorism. Some vegetables can cause gradual suicide or murder in a simple, unsuspected way: potatoes, eggplant, onions with sugar, etc.

Our body consumes energy at the expense of the carbon introduced into our system by our food. The cells, the units of our constitution, destroy and reproduce themselves constantly, always using food for fuel. Life may be considered as a fluid falling through the cellular terrain. The imbalance, which shows itself in the course of this colloid-fall, disappears if one ceases to put in an abnormal nourishment.

The human capacity for resistance, the "terrain of resistance" which is much studied in medicine, as well as the greater part of all illnesses come back to a question of environment, which is to say of nutrition, for this is the way we assimilate our environment into ourselves. In a general way, animals have a greater range (of existence) than vegetation—climatologically and geographically speaking—that hinges solely on this ability. But, once the limit of this ability has been surpassed, even in the place of origin, all animals and humans lose their physiological balance, suffer, and change their very nature. There are some excellent examples presented to us by the biologist M. F. Hoursay. This occurs, by even stronger reason, outside the place of origin. The colonials who returned to Europe every two or three years, but who maintained in the tropical countries their original way of life and nutrition, were in much worse health than the missionaries who remained year after year among the native people, feeding themselves as the natives did.

The Symptom and the Cause

Everything that current medicine considers as a symptom has little importance in traditional Chinese medicine. What was sought was the deep cause of the illness, and neither heredity nor microbes is the cause in this respect.

Study of the disorder is not localized but has bearing on the entire organism, considered as a totality: what has participated at its conception to the present moment, the constitution of the parents (Yin or Yang), the climate the patient has been brought up in and has resided in, and primarily his nutrition, the actual chemical and biological imbalance, etc. . . . It is in this sense that the word "cause" is used, whereas today many symptoms pass for cause.

Classification

There are only two categories of illness.

1. Yin disease, due to an excess of Yin elements.
2. Yang disease, due to an excess of Yang elements.

Or, said otherwise, every illness has two opposite causes. Let us look at myopia, for instance. Yang myopia occurs when the lens is thickened and rounded due to an extreme excess of Yang elements which constrict; whereas Yin myopia is that in which the eye is flattened and elongated due to an excess of dilating Yin elements. These two myopias are completely antithetical as to cause; consequently, they require quite different treatment.

Without this fundamental differentiation, there is no precise therapy. This is why the same X-ray treatment can cure the cancer of one patient and aggravate the cancer of another. This is the inevitable uncertainty of a medicine lacking in true science. First of all, one must determine the Yin or Yang nature of the X-ray and then the Yin or Yang nature of the cancer, according to the case.

All medicine as well as all therapeutic agents also fall into two categories. The Yin ones heal Yang disorders; the Yang ones heal Yin disorders.

But, it must not be taken as a rigid classification from which one might draw up a sort of dictionary. That is why no medicine is more difficult to thoroughly grasp or teach than the ancient Chinese medicine. Yin and Yang classification, as in chemistry, is always relative. The Germans, for example, have given much study to the Chinese medical ordinances, a useless gesture, but, what's more, they have applied them quantitatively, which is even more alarming. The application of doses indicated by the ancient Chinese books could be quite dangerous for Western people, whose biochemical constitution, a direct function of the environment, is altogether different from that of the ancient Chinese. The therapeutic technique of the ancient Japanese doctors is already quite ineffective in many cases in Japan itself, whose inhabitants have changed considerably in their manner of life since their Europeanization.

Besides, the greatest doctors never indicated exact dosages, for this varies according to individual constitution, stage of illness, climate, season, former illnesses, or latest one, etc., and the category in which a certain remedy or a certain illness can be classified is not determined once and for all.

The carp, for example, being animal, is Yang without a doubt in relation to plants. But, as explained in the preceding section, it does not need much oxygen (Yin) and it bears well carbonic gas (CO_2), in the same manner as plants do, and, in actuality, it is very effective in healing Yang cancer, the croup, or Yang pneumonia. The carp is very Yin when compared to other fish, but when well cooked or roasted becomes Yang.

The inflammation of an organ is evidently Yin: But the Yang element, NaCl (salt), for example, which might cause it or the Yang factor, fire, can very well be replaced by ice (Yin). A Yang cause (fire) necessarily produces a Yang condition (heat), but in excess it creates a Yin consequence (inflammation). (Homeopathy, as well as antipathy, must seek their original foundation in these notions.)

Consultation

In keeping with the Oriental concept of cause, which is altogether different from that of Western medicine, medical examination is of necessity synthetic and microscopic. Once the Yin or Yang cause has been determined, the manifestation and localization of the illness are of no great importance, because the symptoms can vary endlessly according to the state, age, and constitution of the sick person, as well as his environment and the season of the year.

The physician must observe the patient in all the aspects of his personality—that is to say, of his biochemical constitution—and then synthesize according to his judgment all that he has seen. The observation of the condition is largely morphological because the form and the shape are determined by the totality of the physical and chemical factors.

Therefore, a physician will observe his patient's eyes, hair, nails, size of ears, voice, gait, handwriting, body, etc.

The pulses are carefully observed, more carefully observed than in present-day medicine.

Therapeutic Technique

No symptomatic or palliative treatments are permitted on principle in traditional Oriental medicine.

1. Operation, amputation, scrapings, etc., are techniques that are scorned as the atrocities committed by an ignorant medical practice that lacks better internal positive treatment.

2. Accessory treatments of an external physical nature, such as moxation, acupuncture, massage, and many other physical treat-

ments unknown in the West, are considered only as a palliative and are only permitted in dire emergencies. Bathing is allowed as a general hygienic accessory. All physical techniques (such as plaster casts, iron braces, packing in ice, etc.) are considered brutal, useless, and even harmful. Hydrotherapy, electrotherapy, radiotherapy, etc., are also palliative and lack flexibility and scientific basis.

3. Serum therapy, vaccination, opotherapy are still palliative. These methods have been known since ancient times.

History is full of examples of people who open their own bodies to give their organs to their loved ones in order to save them.

Medications

All the medications are natural products of such great variety and number that the medical encyclopedia of Li-Che Tohen, published in 1578, consists of 52 volumes.

They are grouped into three categories by their efficiency and manner of action: lowest, middle, and superior.

Those of the lowest group are comparable to those of modern pharmacology, which is to say, they are the most effective in the shortest amount of time but always eventually harmful and dangerous. They are to a point palliative and symptomatic and are only used under very special conditions—to avoid an operation, for example, in a very aged person.

The middle medications are closer to the category of daily food. These are secondary products of the environment and, in general, still a far cry from the superior medications, which are direct products of the natural environment and can heal perfectly. The lower category is only employed temporarily or as accessory. (There is no need to feed glands to a patient in order to cure a diseased gland. The essential cause of the illness is determined and is counter-attacked by direct natural products in a very precise manner.)

The superior medication is daily food with which one can achieve perfect health and happiness.

To sum up, the ancient Chinese medicine considers the living being the transformation of his nutrition and any illness as a phe-

nomenon of imbalance that has occurred in the course of this transformation. Consequently, the medical principle is that every illness
cures itself by a simple adjustment of diet. In practice, the treatment
is also quite simple.

Chinese Physics, Mechanics, and Mathematics

Physics

As we have seen in the Introduction, an isolated science could
not exist in the Orient, or the Oriental spirit. Abstract science, or
scientific teaching, had been assimilated into philosophy from the
time of Fou-Hi.

Ancient people, farmers and shepherds, had no need of science.
They were in possession of the "perfect consciousness" or the "instinct-intuition" (used in the same sense defined previously), which
can be considered analogous to the extremely developed mental
functions of so-called primitive people, such as a perfect sense of
direction, memory, etc., according to Professor Levy-Bruhl.

In fact, one can without much difficulty find all the physical
and mathematical sciences in the ancient Chinese Hindu philosophy
as well as the psychological, economic, and sociological sciences.
But the great men and the emperors guided their people to overlook
and scorn science in order to develop to the end the mental function
which is Perfect Consciousness.

"Scientific knowledge produces a mediocre man, blinded by
shameful desires," Buddha said.

"Your lack of thinking (spontaneity) is the perfect consciousness
taught by your Buddha" said Rinzai.

"Desire for knowledge is a fever," said Lao-tse.

"Learned people have insurmountable difficulties in understanding the Tao, which is easy for the ignorant ones to practice," said
Lao-tse.

A disciple of Confucius was advising a peasant on the use of
a mechanical device (a very simple machine) to draw water from
a well instead of his usual coming-and-going method between the

fields he was irrigating and the stream. The latter replied, "Young man, I thank you for your good advice. But I regret that you have not understood that one must learn through work the true meaning of the Unique Law, the Tao, that one must free oneself from human utilitarian wisdom. Perhaps you are lacking a good teacher, or perhaps your master does not know how to teach the Tao. I am sorry to see this."

Confucius approved of the words of the peasant.

The traditional Japanese architect completely unschooled in physics, geometry, and mathematics, must invent these himself, from the ruler and the Pythagorean theorem to the great law of esthetics, in order to build a five-story pagoda that may be absolutely antiseismic; but he will not preserve by notation the secrets he has discovered in the course of his painful labor, nor will he teach it to his apprentices (see section on Japanese Spirit).

It is evident now that mechanics, mathematics, and physics did not exist in a systematized form. But one must not confuse this apparent neglect of science with the absence of science. Can science actually exist without philosophy? Can philosophy exist without any scientific knowledge? Is not science always governed by instinct? Is not science, which predicts without knowing the cause, only magic? The philosophy that explains the ultimate cause necessarily implies science.

The Prism

The ancient Chinese knew the special scale as well as we do. They used it admirably in biological pentology. They were aware of the physical and physiological effects of all luminous radiations. Had they already invented the prism? If they had arrived at a perfect knowledge of the spectrum without using a prism, we must necessarily admit that their intuitive and instinctive faculties, their mental functions, were extraordinarily developed.

Gravitation

Going by the Unique Law, one can, in principle, establish the law of attraction according to our theory of knowledge and our theory of being. The sixth proposition of the Unique Law teaches us that Yin-Yang activities form aggregates—beings that attract one another. Yin-Yang polarization is of necessity the cause of gravitational force: Yang being the centripetal force; Yin being the centrifugal force. The center of the aggregates necessarily represents the center of attraction. It is a perpetual three-dimensional spiral—not plane, but spherical. The force acts following concentric spheres of surface $\pi(2R)^2$. If the radii of the two spheres are in a ratio of 2 to 1, the forces of attraction would be represented as $1/(4\pi \times 1^2)$ and $1/(4\pi \times 2^2)$ which is 1 to ¼. The force of attraction is, therefore, inversely proportional to the square of the distance.

Atomic Theory of the Proton-nucleus

Professor Tanakadate of the Imperial Academy of Sciences of Japan read my exposition of the spectroscopic classification and informed me that his colleague Professor Nagaoka is very deeply involved in the study of this question. I recently learned that it was Prof. Nagaoka who established the atomic theory of the proton-nucleus. Prior to this, I had considered it as an interpretation of the Unique Law, but I had often asked myself why such a theory had such a peculiar Oriental structure. I believe that Prof. Nagaoka, as well as his very old friend Prof. Tanakadate, during his childhood approximately 70 years ago—the period when traditional education was in full bloom in Japan—had studied the four books and five ching, the Canons of *In'yology*. After long years of scientific research, he returned to his childhood—the Unique Law—due not to science, but to his "consciousness," which had once been cultivated by traditional education. Unconsciously, he picked up the Unique Law in the very modern guise of a physicist. Perhaps I have made an error in attributing this theory to Prof. Nagaoka, but my own mistake would bring me still greater happiness, for it would prove to me that certain Oriental spirits are capable of a conception of the world and of matter analogous to that of the science of the Far-East.

Astronomy and Geometry
I have nothing to add to what Prof. A. Rey has written in Volume IV of *Science Orientale dans L'Antiquite*. On the contrary, I have found there a great number of notions that I was missing before.

Mathematics and Mechanics
Once one has learned the accomplishments of the ancient Chinese—that they foresaw eclipses, observed the black spots on the sun (their periodicity and influence on the universe), already knew the function of various intensities of the respiratory system, had measured accurately the rate of motion of blood circulation (they performed difficult operations, or at least difficult for the modern surgeon, such as the opening of the breast and abdominal cavity), could distinguish by auscultation the particular sound of each organ (the stomach, lungs, heart, liver, kidneys, etc.), manufactured a great many weapons (varied and rather advanced of design), and erected magnificent palaces and citadels—it is not difficult to imagine that their mathematical and mechanical knowledge was developed along practical lines. Their astronomy, the logic that is portrayed in their symbolic, ideographic, and graphic characters—a written language common to all the Chinese people—is worthy of admiration, and it proves to us without any doubt a logical and mathematical superiority.

Their rather advanced mathematical knowledge is confirmed by such evidence as:

1. The Sticks of Logos, which interpret phenomena by two distinct ideological categories: the first one implies exclusively chronological causality; the second one implies a causality of space. (The complete study of the permutation of these two complex causalities into 64 symbols and the most complex laws, which define the relationship between these symbols; the interpretation of the significant character of each stick within these 64 symbols, which amounts to 384 defining symbols.)

2. The 50 bamboo or yarrow stalks that are the traditional preparation for forecasting.

3. Later inventions of various calculating tools, such as the 200 small sticks in Japan (which allow us to extract the square or cubic root), as well as various types of abacuses, which are so practical that I use them instead of arithmetical tables or the slide rule.

The Japanese bow, more than two meters long, has some remarkable aspects from the physical and mechanical point of view, as well as the Japanese saber, which, however, is relatively modern. The metal of the latter contains a delicate proportion of molybdenum; they were always manufactured in the mountains far removed from the seashore (the conditions are very important—in this case, an abundance of Yin activities) by masters who rigorously observed the particular physiological laws according to the ruling *Shin do fu ji* and were always made of amorphous limonite (Fe_3O_4) of whose industrial use modern science has no knowledge. Their curve, their particular metallurgic construction, which deadens the conductivity of violent shocks to the hand, etc., surpass ordinary physical and mechanical science.

Climatology

The *Canon of the Emperor Houang-Ti* reports lengthy animated discussions between minister-philosophers and scientists, which forced the emperor to declare an end—a halt without recorded conclusion—to the diverse opinions on scientific questions. One of these remarkable discussions is of the physiological and medical determination into four levels or four natures of foods and medications: extreme Yang, moderate Yang, moderate Yin, extreme Yin. Let us leave this aside. But the geographical determination of these four climatological degrees is very important in the natural sciences and their applications.

It was for this reason that the great Japanese scientific spirit Ishizuka Sagen, founder of the school of the Renaissance of Traditional Medicine (the origin of today's Society of Traditional Medicine), recognized the public usefulness of the Unique Law and made a proposition 50 years ago to modern science that they modify the customary five zones into eight zones: two tropical; two cool, two temperate, and two cold. This division is the physical and biological translation of the Unique Law. It is very important in biology, in medicine, in history, in economic geography. The distribution of plants and animals, the races, the physical and moral differences between races, etc., are related to it.

My teacher, Mr. Nishibata, clearly defined four zones of 22.5°, each on the two sections of the earth divided by the equator. I have modified them to do away with the rigidity of such a division by substituting for them the three irregular homeothermal lines encircling the globe that indicate the three average temperatures: 68°, 40°, 32° Fahrenheit.

To conclude, I do not think that the Orient should take pride in the antiquity of its philosophy. Neither tradition nor novelty are signs of superiority. The philosophy of the Orient is a necessary by-product, due entirely and simply to its biological environment, and the same holds true for Oriental science. The Orient, mother of the philosophy of *Shunyata,* is a sunny land, warm and gay; whereas, the cradle of the dazzling extroverted science is closed, somber, and sad. History is the biological translation of geography.

The Spirit of the Oriental People

In order to conclude our brief studies, we shall finally examine what has taken place during the past 2500 or 3000 years in the philosophy and science of the Far-East, and at what stage the Chinese, Hindu, and Japanese spirits have arrived in the 20th century.

The Chinese Spirit

The Chinese people are the representatives of the oldest positivist philosophy in the world. Their philosophy, as we have already seen, is based on scientific research conducted for centuries. It betrays no superstitions, religions, nor mystical element in its origin. It was altogether practical. It did not personify the idea of creation in a personal god. It named the Unique Law that rules the world "the Sky" (the Sun), but this does not refer to the physical sky that we understand today. This philosophy succeeded in creating a spiritual body of teachings of universal value that governed people for a long time, until the time of Confucius. Its form of writing, the most philosophic and symbolic in the world, shows qualities of intuition, synthesis, and an extraordinarily practical spirit to those who study it deeply in its original form. It connected and unified all the Chinese people dispersed over the whole continent of central Asia, speaking diverse languages, during the prehistoric period. It was the common written language. (According to Li-Ki, the population at that time was almost 308,000,000.)

Chinese pragmatism was developing through the written word (ideograph); astronomy, mathematics, industry, and, above all, physiology were being perfected when decadence overtook the pragmatic spirit. Midway in this disintegration, philosophers—Confucius, Lao-tse, etc.—struggled to safeguard the happiness of the people.

Confucius was much more modern in thought than Lao-tse. They both preached the same ancient philosophy, but Confucius was detached from it, whereas Lao-tse actually lived it. It was only at the age of 50 that Confucius began his serious study of the *I-Ching*, which he continued until his death. Before that time, he had taught a sort of moral code, a set of obligatory rulings of convention. In that sense, Lao-tse was much his superior because he applied solely the ancient philosophy of Fou-Hi taken from the *I-Ching*.

At one time, it is said, Confucius was strongly criticized and reproached by Lao-tse, but he listened to the criticism and accepted all of it. Upon his return, one of his disciples asked him what he thought of Lao-tse.

Confucius replied, "I am not astonished when I see birds fly, fish swim, and four-legged animals run. I know that fish are caught in nets, and four-legged animals in traps, and that one stops short the flight of birds with arrows. But as for the Dragon, I do not know how he can be borne by the winds and the clouds and rise into the sky. Today, I have seen Lao-tse; he resembles the Dragon."

Confucius' doctrine was necessarily far removed from the original one. He died at the age of 70.

While he was making an intense study of the *I-Ching,* he said, "I have finally reached a stage where obeying one's desires is not in violation of the law."

This is the world where there is no need to force oneself to conform to numerous conventional rules. It is the world of *Taikyoku*, the universe of *Shunyata* and of Tao. It is an ideal world that does not require any human artifice; it is the philosophy of spontaneity where everything is perfect.

"Virtue is light as a feather that follows every wind. It is on every occasion delicate and exquisite. But it still is accomplished by a trace of contrivance, just as a feather still has some weight, however imperceptible. Tao, the Unique Law (*Shunyata*), has no weight, no sound. It embraces and directs the entire universe." This Confucius stated when he finally reached the Tao after long years of devoted attention to the *I-Ching*.

Among the sayings of Lao-tse are the following:

"The only thing which I fear is to act" (following the dictates of the small "self" and not of the Unique Law).

"Struggle against the fever of knowing all."

"It is by the absence of thought and reflection (knowledge) that one can learn about the Tao...the inactive word is correct, and opinionated folly is not far from it. However, he who knows does not speak; he who speaks knows nothing. That is the reason why the wise man follows the system of silence. There is no other way to follow the Tao; there is no other way to achieve virtue...."

"Ceremony is mutual hypocrisy."

"Consequently, one might say: when the Tao was lost, it was replaced by justice; when justice was lost, it was replaced by ceremony. Ceremony is the last blooming (which is to say, the last degeneration) of the Tao and the principle of disorder."

"Man (Yang) is fed and governed by the Earth (Yin); the Earth is governed by the Sky (Yang, the Sun); the Sky is governed by the Tao and the Tao is governed by the Highest Nature (*Taikyoku*)," said Lao-tse.

Tao is the Unique Law—Nature. A simple peasant who pays absolute obedience to nature understands this and is happy, enjoying a long and peaceful life.

The tireless and obstinate scholar, seeking to know all and making determined efforts to find out the fundamental laws, may very well end up without knowing the Tao.

The philosophy of the Far-East is a Macrobiotic way of life, simple and easy to follow for the uneducated, but almost impossible to understand for a scientist; just like the difference in the rate of mortality among peasants, on the one hand, and physicians and biologists on the other.

These two great monuments to humanity, the teaching of Confucius and the teaching of Lao-tse, half destroyed by wars, covered over by moss and weeds—are they now abandoned? The ancient philosophy of Fou-Hi—is it forgotten?

No! Despite the injuries of time and the wear and tear of centuries, the entire philosophy and its teaching still exist because of their simplicity and absolute superiority. If Western civilization and the material or spiritual colonization that comes with it can reach China, it will be assimilated in *Taikyoku* some day, just as fire (symbol of material civilization), violent as it is, rises and disappears into the air, the great Yin.

Referring to the future of China, the first august ruler Fou-Hi said simply, *"Ten ko ken"* (the evolution of the Tao is perfect!). This is the first sentence that we shall meet in the *I-Ching*. If we wish to find out what the present state of China has in store, it would show the "Sin" of the Sticks of Logos: ☷. Here is the Dragon, sleeping under the ground. Above him, the crowd dances, fights, weeps. Woe to the Westerners who don't know it. The Dragon sleeps!

The Hindu Spirit

India is a very Yang country. All year long, the sun scorches the land. Consequently, that which grows there, in order to absorb such intense heat, has to be very Yin. That is why there is such luxurious vegetation in all of India. Fruits, extremely rich in K (index of Yin activity) are in abundance as well as other yin produce, which constitutes the diet of the population. Because it is so extremely hot, it is virtually impossible to work fast and energetically; one is forced to be calm. The Hindu philosophy is, therefore, necessarily meditative, withdrawing from the subtle differentiations of the relative world, hiding in cool forests.

The Hindus thus arrived at the philosophy of Brahma or of *Shunyata (Ku* in Chinese or Japanese). The paths that have led them to this achievement are entirely different from those of the Chinese, but both end at the same high point, although philosophical schools, religions, and sects are numerous in India, and some of them appear to contradict others.

Shunyata: This is the sound of the whole Hindu philosophy, as well as the whole philosophy of the Far-East. It is very difficult to understand, especially for Westerners. When it is literally translated as the "Void" or "Emptiness," its spirit is almost impossible to grasp. Perhaps, after long studies, some will understand this concept of *Shunyata*, but they will not be able to feel it in reality. How many Japanese understand it through the Chinese translation *Ku*? I don't know.

The one who understands it perfectly must live it himself, and in no other way must he live: he is a Buddha. The knowledge of *Synnyata, Ku, Tao,* or *Taikyoku* is worthless. One will never understand these various names without finding oneself at the very center of the Law of Nature. It is not through "knowledge" as we have defined it, but in "consciousness" that one can grasp *Shunyata*.

The more one studies *Shunyata* in numerous books, the further one removes oneself from it. The more analytical or modern one is in spirit, the less is one capable of understanding it.

Originally, there were no differences between the Hindu and the Chinese philosophy. They drifted apart from each other due to the contrasting environments in which they developed. The differentiation was already noticeable at the time of Confucius and Shakyamuni. The Hindu philosophy was purely philosophical, meditative, and mystical, while that of the Chinese was pragmatic and scientific. It was a necessary consequence of the opposite characters of the two nations: one represented the cold Yin continent north of the highest mountains, the other the warm country south of the same mountains. One went in the direction of a national morality, the other to a religion.

The theory of knowledge, for example, is much more developed in India than in China, as well as that of "being." The books dealing with it are countless. The Hindu logic is altogether unique. That which corresponds to the Greek syllogism makes up three, four, or five propositions in reverse order:

1st proposition: There is a fire in the mountain.

2nd proposition: Because there is smoke a resulting "phenomenon."

3rd proposition: Just as in the hearth, for example.

It is the intuition that acts in the Hindu logic; that is to say, this logic reproduces the order of our understanding in daily life.

Psychology, medicine, and physiology were extremely well developed in India in antiquity, and with a much more philosophical approach than even in China. Consequently, they are much more difficult to understand than the latter; modern people have no understanding of the ancient Chinese medicine. All the more, no one can grasp the ancient Hindu medical science. It is curious that we meet (in Japan) priests or Buddhist philosophers who are themselves ill! They still want to save the world, just as the ancient Buddhists, but don't know how to save themselves! Can Buddhism, which cannot cure physical sickness, cure spiritual sickness, which is continuous with the small "self?" Only those who live it physiologically can understand such a philosophy.

As in China, all of science is unified by philosophy. The latter is a Macrobiotic way, or rather, it is beyond Macrobiotics: Nirvana, eternal life, life within *Shunyata.*

The priests of every Hindu religion, just as the Chinese philosophers, were obligated to know medicine; thus, the ideal administration written of by A. Comte was realized. The priests not only saved souls from spiritual miseries but also from physical anguish.

The transcendental superiority of the ancient medicine of India and China was apparent in the life histories of the great priests and the great philosophers, in their health, their tranquility, their self-possession, and their imperceptible but constant smile—the reflection of superior satisfaction. It is said that Shakyamuni died at the age of 80. A life of 80 years in a country where all the living beings mature very early is remarkable; it equals a life of 100 years or more in a more temperate climate. Shinran died at the age of 90 years, after having spent a life of difficulties.

Shakyamuni synthesized all the religions of prehistoric India into

Buddhism, whose original spirit almost no longer exists in the Hindu Buddhism of today. But we can also consider the original Buddhism as representing all ancient religions, because it does not contain any new element. Having said this, let us meditate profoundly on what it teaches: *Amida, Karma, Goun* (the five elements), and *Shunyata*. We find *Shunyata* is the exact equivalent of *Taikyoku*; *Amida* is identical to the personified *Tao*; *Goun* to the aggregations of the two fundamental activities; and *Karma* is nothing but the dynamic law regulating Yin and Yang. Thus, by *In'yology* we modern and analytical degenerates will understand Buddhism a little more easily and, thus, all Hindu philosophy.

Amida possesses many names: *Miroku, Nyorai, Shinnyo, Ichinyo*, etc. All these signify "That which appears present," "That which appears absent," "The eternal light," etc. One can clearly see its relationship with the *Tao* and *Taikyoku*, which we have studied in Part 2.

Following the death of Shakyamuni, Buddhism divided itself into two fundamental sects: *Mahayana* (Great Buddhism) and *Hinayana* (Small Buddhism). The first is much more philosophical and religious; the second much more moral. By "religious," we mean that which directs us toward the perfect freedom of *Taikyoku, Shunyata*. By "moral," we mean that which brings us to the limited freedom of the small "self" (according to the theory of knowledge of the Far-East).

These two fundamental sects ramified endlessly in India, China, and Japan throughout the centuries. Mahayana Buddhism disappeared from India and China and was imported into Japan from China approximately a dozen centuries ago. It developed there well and still remains active. One will see it clearly by reading the words of Shinran (see the first Appendix).

Along with Buddhism, a great number of Sanscrit words were introduced into the Chinese and Japanese languages. But no equivalent philosophy, no Chinese science was introduced into India at the same time. Linguists and historians are mute on this point. Some do state that this is due to the inferiority of the then existing Chinese and Japanese civilizations. But the Chinese philosophy, already perfected long before the time of Confucius was as ancient as the Hindu philosophy and its spirit was identical.

Others say that the Chinese who migrated to India at this time were ignorant merchants. I do not believe that the ancient Chinese were all so egotistical and materialistic. Some students and Chinese men of science did go to India; furthermore, several Hindu Buddhist priests came to China and remained there quite a long time.

My opinion on this point is simple enough. The philosophy conceived in India—a warm country, Yang, under a burning sun— aimed inevitably at the coolness of the shade in the virgin forest, at tranquility, at the deepest contemplation, at all that is most Yin. Conversely, the philosophy born in the central plateau of China—in the dead center of the Yin cold—had the sun, the sky, great warmth, power, energy, matter, as an ideal. It was, therefore, Yang. The Chinese people were active and open to everything; they welcomed with open arms the Hindu philosophy. But being pragmatic and materially oriented, they finally abandoned Buddhism. The Hindus, on the contrary, were resigned, retiring, hiding, refusing light and heat, meditating in the coolness of the primeval forests. They did not even want to imagine heat, activity, energy, and movement in the Chinese manner. Consequently, they could not accept even the least part of the rather scientific philosophy of China, although the latter was the twin spirit of their own. The situation is being repeated today in relation to the materialistic civilization of the West. It is unbearable for the Hindus. No amount of enforcement will ever succeed in this importation—the history of 30 centuries proves it. One must stop disturbing the contemplation of the extremely modest, humble Hindus, worshipers of the tranquil virgin forests. If the ancient Chinese pragmatism was rejected by them, with even stronger reason so will be modern scientific civilization.

The present state of the Hindu people can be represented by the symbol *Hi* (obstruction): ☶☷.

The force of ascent, Yin symbol *Kon* ☷ is crushed by the weight, Yang *Ken* ☶. The oppression cannot be a lasting condition.

The Japanese Spirit

I am not referring to the Japan of today. Except for old traditional families, Japan has lost the true Oriental spirit. It has retained only an Americanized Russian Salad of Communism and Capitalism, of movies and jazz. Never having rediscovered an equilibrium outside the one it has abandoned, modern Japan has no interest for us at the moment.

Ancient Japan had no metaphysics, no science, no moral religion, morality, nor any concepts such as Heaven or Hell. It was and still is a land of people dwelling in understanding. The *Kojiki* (a history of antiquity dating back more than 1200 years) proves it. It is a natural history of the creation of the universe, of long journeys and adventure across the oceans, which the ancestral Japanese performed in prehistoric times. (Shintoism is but a national cult of the ancestors, nothing more.) Their sole interest was practical living; it is, therefore, realism that directed the Japanese people, from its origin to the present. Let us summarily examine what this Japanese realism consists of.

It is justly said that the Japanese people are the cleverest imitators in the world of Western civilizations. When more than fifteen hundred years ago contact was made with the Chinese civilization for the first time, the Japanese took from it all it had to offer: the alphabet and script, philosophy, Taoism, Buddhism, literature, the arts and trades, the costumes, etc. They refused nothing.

For a period of 60 years, the Japanese persisted in a complete importation of Western civilization. They even exaggerated it.

To accept everything and leave nothing unexplored, nothing foreign, is the true Japanese spirit. It is a little too enamored of all that is new. It practices everything before judging. It believes nothing can spoil it; it has every confidence in the Great Will of Amida.

But the *Nembutsuist* is much more a vegetarian than the converted vegetarian (ex-carnivore or reactionary) of other countries. Besides, he is more emotionally sensitive; he has no indifference even toward vegetal life. He knows how to greet a turnip when taking a leaf from it; he will pick up grains spilled on the road one by one, clean them with care, revere them as Buddha, and bring them home. "Rice is Buddha" says a Japanese proverb.

One should see the revelation of the Great Will of Amida in each grain of rice. Such is the Japanese teaching of Butsudo.

All general traditional education aims at the perfect comprehension of the Unique Law by the most varied roads. All the daughters of Buddhist or traditional families learn various arts such as *Shodo* (the *Do* of writing), *Gado* (the *Do* of painting), *Kado* (the *Do* of poetry), *Geido* (the *Do* of music or song of the poetical classical dance), etc., and esthetic practices such as *Kado* (the *Do* of flowers), *Sado* (the *Do* of tea), etc. All of them make up part of the one *Do*, the synthesizing Japanese culture, that makes its people decipher the Unique and Fundamental Law through all of these various arts.

Sado is well explained in the *Book of Tea* by Okakura, which has several French translations. All the cultured samurais of other days learned the tea ceremony, and the traditional Japanese even today learns and observes it. Its teaching is not limited to girls.

Kado (or *Shikishima No Michi*) is an esthetic synthesis that teaches us how to improve our comprehension, our admiration of the Great Will through natural phenomena, or in every scene of our daily life by the *Waka* (poems in 31 syllables).

Kado (the ritual of flowers) teaches how to arrange plants, leaves, or flowers of all sorts in the most esthetic manner possible with the least number of cuttings—the plants are alive!—and how to make them live as long as possible in a certain pose, in a combination both artistic and altogether natural so that each leaf and each flower might receive light perfectly, allowing us in this way to admire the graciously caught image of the Great Supernatural Will.

The education of boys has the same spirit.

Judo (*Jujitsu*) is a dynamic physical culture, a practical science and synthesis of the *In'yological* physiology and philosophy.

Kendo (fencing), *Kyudō* (archery) are also typical. Foreigners, as well as modern Japanese, confuse them with sports; it is lamentable.

Bushido or *Shido* (the *Do* of the samurais or of traditional Japanese) has already been vaguely known in Europe for a long time.

Ido (the *Do* of Oriental medicine), which I have treated in "Chinese Medicine," aims at eliminating medicine entirely.

If a man has once been saved by Oriental medicine, he has no possibility of falling ill again in his lifetime. Otherwise, he has not been truly cured, or he has not grasped the essence of this medical practice. If he becomes ill several times again, he is not worth curing. He must be allowed to suffer that he might learn the law. This is saving him in reality and is the only way of doing so. The Unique Law wishes it thus for natural selection and to consolidate the happiness of all of humanity.

One shouldn't treat the sickness itself; it is useless; the sickness is variable. It has its wonderful faculty of adaptation. One must create the constitution, then ground the inner environment so soundly that the factors of the disease cannot penetrate into it or are no longer active in it. This is the perfect physiological synthesis, which all animals possess instinctively. Let us not confuse this with preventative medicine, which is but another applied analytic science. The perfect medicine, the *Ido*, is the medical synthesis of all the *In'yological* knowledge of the entire universe.

Kado, the *Do* of poetry, as interpreted by the *Haiku*, is a poem in 17 syllables: 5, 7, and again 5. It is forbidden to express it with an ephemeral human emotion. It reveals an exquisite world where there is no sadness, no sorrow. It is the absolute world where all is good and beautiful, where all is to be admired and thanked. There is no place in it for sentimentality. If one is not happy, it is because one lacks poetic gifts and understanding of the Unique Law—one lacks modesty and faith.

Here is a poem by Issa (1752-1817), for example:

> *Taku hodo wa kaze ga mote kuru ochiba kana!*
> "The wind brings me
> as many dry leaves

as I have need
of for the fire."

You see that here no word expresses sentiment. It is a simple sketch. A poet lives alone in a remote part of the country or in a dale surrounded by mountains. He reaps the dead leaves that the wind pushes there morning and evening when he has need of them, either to cook his rice or to heat his hut. He is always content with the great benevolence of Amida, who is his protector. Without a sense of Japanese Buddhism, its poetry cannot be understood.

As I have often said previously, the majority of the great samurais believed in Amida. Often the flags that they carried into the battlefields bore the name of Buddha. They did not go to war to kill their enemies but to die a splendid death as faithful warriors for their masters or their emperor, to go to the Great Joy of Amida, the world of *Shunyata*, as soon as possible. Now it will be clear why and in what spirit the samurais improvised their last poems before committing hara-kiri or dying in a hand-to-hand struggle on the battlefield. They paid their respects to their enemies, each according to his station, with the same ceremony they gave to their partisans. The one who is dying says, "*Namu Amida Butsu.*" All those surrounding him also say it. The two samurais—the winner and the loser—also repeat this phrase, even the one who is condemned to death.

The *Nembutsu* is also equivalent to a greeting: "Farewell. In the Great Joy! My friends, my enemies, we shall all be happy in *Shunyata, Namu Amida Butsu!*"

All of the Hindu or Chinese philosophy, which has been imported into Japan, developed, modified, perfected, still exists in other forms in the entire Japanese body of knowledge: Mahayana Buddhism in *Butsudo*, Chinese medicine in *Ido*, Chinese philosophy in *Bushido* and *Shido*, Chinese physiology in *Sado, Kado, and Shokuyodo*, etc... But these *Dos* are not written about.

Japanese Buddhism has no canon of its own. Shintoism has no book comparable to the Bible. There is a book of *Bushido*. No commentary can explain the Japanese spirit. It is too lively to be grasped by dead words. It explains itself everywhere and at all times. There is no strictly Japanese writing, not even today. Although there are some fifty characters (Japanese syllabaries), they are never employed independently.

The ancient Japanese did not want to transform their land into a "land of letters," but they were very proud of their *Yamato*—land of the Gods, happy and superior land in possession of a marvelous language (which does not require a written script because it is so simple and systematic).

It is exactly the same spirit possessed by Fou-Hi, who was satisfied with his three Sticks of Logos to interpret all phenomena of the entire universe, all the philosophy, all the science and all the national body of teachings. The more one uses these words and letters, the further one removes oneself from the spirit, the Unique Law.

The uselessness of all teachings of the ways is understood. These ways are not considered to be indispensable. One dwells on perfecting the consciousness, the instinct-intuition.

Japanese poetry is characteristic of this nation. It is a simple and naive esthetic expression of the knowledge of the Unique Law; it is the voice of consciousness. It has an unpretentious form of 17 or 31 syllables because it dares not spoil the representation of intimate nature by useless words.

In the same vein, Japanese painting does not intend to represent all details, but rather through any form, intimate nature itself—*Shunyata, Taikyoku*.

The more one tampers with it, the more obscure this deepest nature becomes. This spirit is not altogether lost even in the common wood-block prints of Utamaro. But the true monocolored (black and white) painting of Japan is not easy to understand in the sense that the essence of nature is explained in it. One must grasp the imperceptible *Shunyata* behind the brush strokes.

Mannyoshu, the first anthology of Japanese poetry (edited under the direction of the emperor in the Nara Period at the beginning of the 8th century), shows us explicitly that *Kado* (the *Do* of poetry) was the national teaching. It comprises more than 5000 poems (*Tanka* and *Tyoka*, not *Haiku*) written by emperors, samurais, officers of the army, dignitaries, empresses and princesses, common girls, soldiers, beggars, and so on. In other words, it represents the entire nation. No one was called "poet" or "poetess," but everyone was one. It is the ideal of the Japanese spirit. He who does not have his consciousness freed from insignificant knowledge could not compose poems of 17 or 31 syllables.

Emperor Meiji, who died about twenty years ago, was a great poet. Even today, at each new year, the emperor receives innumerable poems from the entire nation. But neither now nor in the past was there a school of rhetoric, esthetics, or poetry.

Haiku is a derivation of ancient Japanese poetry. Its founder was Basho. One day, he was receiving his friend, a Buddhist priest. The conversation was almost wordless because words lose touch with deep friendship. A nearly silent visit is quite sufficient for those who can grasp everything through their clairvoyant instinct-intuition.

"The Unique Law, before the advent of moss—what was it?" asked the priest, while gazing into the pond of Basho's moss-covered garden. The poet did not answer . . .

A low sound, almost imperceptible, vibrated through and unified the silence. It was a frog jumping into the pond.

Both priest and poet were motionless.

"A noise in water made by a frog, wasn't it?" replied Basho. He had sketched out *Taikyoku* with an imperceptible sound produced in the water, which dies out in the surrounding silence. He had interpreted the depth of the sea of *Taikyoku* by the silence, and the ephemeral beings that die out and return endlessly unto the ether-universe by this brief noise, which in the same way dies out into the infinite. And this meant, in replying to his guest, that the Unique Law in the prehistoric world where the vegetation of moss had not yet appeared was as ungraspable as the sound that had vanished.

"The sound of a frog in the water—how marvelous! Thank you," murmured the priest, satisfied.

An old pond
A frog jumps in the
Water—sound

This is one of the best-known poems of Basho. The translation loses the nobility and simplicity of the style that is characteristic of the philosophy of intuition.

Haiku is at the very heart of the universe, *Shunyata*, where there is no trace of beings, no sentiment, no objectivity, nor subjectivity; it is beyond sentiment, knowledge, humanity, and mundane compassion.

One day the poet, journeying on foot and following a solitary road near a river, crossed a vast beach covered with tall reeds. He stopped suddenly, hearing some disturbance. It was a very small infant abandoned, no doubt due to poverty, crying in a basket. He looked at him and hesitated. He remained on the spot for a few instances, and finally departed after having made a *numbutsu*. Few persons would dare to act this way; our small "compassion" would not allow us. But the poet of *Shunyata* does not sell compassion cut-rate. He is too great to receive an individual soul. He embraces all humanity. Neither the death nor the life of ephemeral beings bind him. For the poet of *Taikyoku*, all beings are the continuity of his own existence, just as this child was. By going away, he succeeded in resigning himself to the fragile world of the beings. It was he himself that he was abandoning in the reeds; his existence had no importance for him, nor had it for a long time, because he had entered into the real being *Shunyata*. He always said to his disciples that each of his poems was his last farewell to the world.

Everyone likes *Haiku* or *Waka*. But there is no public education for *Haiku*, which is simple and easy to learn. There is no difficulty in arranging words in the order of 5, 7, 5 syllables. But to arrive at the highest stage of *Haiku*, all depends on the consciousness, on the faculty that contemplates the intimate nature in all of creation.

Each poem, each *Haiku*, is an esthetic and intuitive expression of phenomena evolving both in nature and in human society.

An unknown Japanese architect said, "When I was 25 years old, I built a five-story pagoda. I had difficulties, I worried very much, I made extraordinary efforts. I felt myself dying. It was, in fact, more painful than death. I declared that when I finished the work, I would never again attempt such a task. At the age of 40, however, I did start again. It was no less painful than the first time. When it was completed, I declared that it would be my last accomplishment in this world. But at the age of 50, I had to begin once more, and I found still more difficulties. I said to myself, I must sacrifice my life to achieve this work. If I should die the day following the erection of the building, I would not regret it. . . . It always seemed to me that the pagodas were built by someone other than myself. . ."

The Japanese pagoda, made entirely of wood, is without equal in architectural design for resisting earthquakes. The principal pillar is suspended to counterbalance the shocks (vibrations). There are some pagodas in existence that date back more than a thousand years. The Hindu pagoda—golden, glass ornamented, sparkling in the equatorial light of India—is magnificent but incapable of tolerating the smallest shock.

The decoration and esthetic composition of the entire design of the Japanese pagoda depends, now as before, on an architect ignorant of geometry, physics, the art of design, and mathematics because the traditional architect does not receive any formal training. He must invent everything himself.

Once the work has begun, he no longer eats in the way in which he is accustomed. He removes himself from his wife. He is as if divinely possessed. His instinct-intuition alone is working with extraordinary vigor. This is the Japanese technique of education. The result is not the *raison d'etre* because it is the faculty of seizing the consciousness of *Taikyoku* of *Shunyata* that is aimed for; the pagoda is only a souvenir of it, just as *Haiku* or *Waka*.

To sum up, the Japanese spirit is a realism that does away with all subtle discussions, all partial teachings, all philosophy, all science, by melting them and assimilating them into practical life in an esthetic manner. It does not allow specializations or specialists.

It asks only for ordinary natural men who strive to have a clear and precise instinct-intuition, the consciousness of *Shunyata*. The true Japanese must be simple in his life, intuitive and instinctive in practice but never diplomatic.

Conclusion

1. The principle of philosophy and science is identical at its origin in China, India, and Japan. It is *Shunyata, Taikyoku,* or *Ku,* which more or less interpret the true universe.

2. The Unique Principle evolved towards pragmatism in China. It continues to guide the whole nation.

3. The Unique Principle developed into a religious form in India. This was the indispensable form for the Hindu.

4. In Japan, it melted into the practical daily life and became the Japanese spirit, which also assimilated the philosophy of India and China.

5. The practical Chinese spirit will reform New China little by little. It will not accept all of the Western civilization.

6. The Hindu philosophy will end up in a renewed civilization, particularly spiritual. It will refuse modern civilization.

7. One day Japan will also return to its tradition—at the same time keeping the materialistic European civilization—and will finally forge it and assimilate it into its practical daily life. It will remain the most Europeanized in the Orient.

8. The ancient Chinese philosophy and science will be studied by Westerners, but not by the Japanese, Chinese, or Hindus. They will be found still alive, still applicable, and much will be gained from them.

This is the divining symbol that explains the conflict between the Western civilization and the quiet one of *Shunyata.*

93

Tannishyo
(Regret for Foreign Belief)

The Words of Shinran Recorded by His Disciple

Preface

As I meditate on the past and the present, I regret to see people drifting away from the true belief of our Sect, the belief that Shinran, our teacher, explained so well. I fear these people are lost and are experiencing only doubts and difficulties.

It is impossible to enter into the Easy Way if a person has not, through good fortune, found sages and followed their instruction.

Let not reason weaken the belief in the Easy Way!

Thus, I am writing these lines, those words of our teacher Shinran that still remain with me, not only to clear up some difficult problems but also to guide our friends to the Easy Way.

Vocabulary

Amida, Amida-Buddha: The greatest spirit of Buddhism: not an imaginary existence nor a concept, but the unique, true, and eternal existence that directs humanity and all that exists according to a perfect harmony. Another term of *Amida* is *Tao*. A stands for *Taikyoku*, infinity, or inner nature; *Mi*, beings; *Da*, the law that assimilates the latter into the former. (See Chapter 2 of the *Unique Principle*.)

Nembutsu: *Nem*, contemplation; *Butsu*, Amida Buddha, *Nembutsu*, the contemplation of Amida Buddha; the expression of eternal gratitude.

Karma: Universal determinism.

Namu Amida Butsu!: Mute or expressed calling forth to the great spirit of all existence. The appellation is implicit; the contemplation is explicit: that is the sole principle of the True Sect, Shin Sect, *Shinshu*, the Sect of Nembutsu. *Namu* signifies: Oh! Wonderful. *Namu Amida Butsu:* Oh! Wonderful great Amida Buddha!

Shinran: Disciple of Honen. He founded the Shinshu Sect or the True Sect. Through his words, one can clearly see that Buddhism is a religion created for the most corrupt, the most lamentable, and the most dishonest. It wasn't created for respectable people or for scholars because it isn't a system of morals but a true religion. If morals are based on the small "self," on the infinitesimal individual, religion is based on the true universe. (Always according to the theory of knowledge.)

Easy Way: The True Sect receives and saves everyone unconditionally; everyone can enter it and achieve his goal. Thus, it is called the Easy Way. The Easy Way to happiness, that is to say, live in eternal gratitude for Amida Buddha who gives up his Buddhahood if there is a single person who lives in unhappiness in this world.

The Great Joy, the Supreme Joy: This is the perfect and eternal world of *Taikyoku, Shunyata,* or Inner Nature.

Chapter 1

How wonderful and grateful I feel when I recognize Amida's Supreme Will. When one has the intention of thus practicing Nembutsu while meditating, he finds himself already happily received into the hands of Great Amida, who protects us eternally and who abandons no one. The Great Will of Amida never distinguishes the honest from the dishonest nor the young from the old. Only faith is important. To save the most dishonest, the most pitiful, the most sensuous, and the most impure is the Great Will of Amida.

Chapter 2

The Master Shinran speaks to scholars on a pilgrimage: "Fortunately, you have arrived here across countries and mountains risking your lives to ask me the means of acquiring Supreme Joy. (The voyage was extremely difficult and dangerous during this feudal period.)

"But, unfortunately, if you think that I know some means other than Nembutsu to arrive at the Great Joy, or know of special and sacred documents, you are mistaken.

"If you wish to learn of them, you have only to go see the scholars of the City of the South (Nara) or of the Mountain of the North (Hiei).

"I know of nothing more than Nembutsu. According to my master, you have only to do Nembutsu to be saved by Amida. There you have my faith. There is nothing else.

"Is Nembutsu really the key that permits us to enter into the Sublime World, or is it an act that makes us fall into Hell? Of that I am completely ignorant.

"Even if we are deceived by our master, Honen, and fall into Hell, we should not repent.

"Because we completely lack the capacity to accomplish one act or another that would bring us unfailingly to Buddha, we are destined only to Hell. Let us reflect deeply on this. (We believe the contrary because of the same mentality that makes us think ourselves wise. To do a moral act is egotism; not the true good at all. Morality is a collection of conventional regulations between egotistical animals.)

"If the Will of Amida is true, the word of Shakyamuni Buddha is not false; if the word of Shakyamuni Buddha is true, the teaching of Zendo can only be true. If the teaching of Zendo is true, the explanation of Honen is just. And, finally, if the explanation of Honen is just, what Shinran says is not a lie.

"After all, this is my faith.

"Now, you have only to take Nembutsu or leave it; you are completely free."

Chapter 3

"If even the honest can be saved, why not the dishonest?"

But people are always saying the contrary: "If even the dishonest can be saved, why not the honest?"

At first glance, that seems very reasonable, but it is a strange reasoning and understands nothing of the Will of Amida. The honest person, proud of his independence of will, his capacity to do good, and his honesty, necessarily lacks submission and absolute confidence toward the Will of Amida. He does not like to recognize that he is directed and protected by something outside of himself. When he abandons the petty pride of his honesty and faithfully follows the Will of Amida, he can enter into the Great Joy.

By birth we are sensuous, vain, dishonest, impure, incapable of doing the slightest good whatever it may be, and always enclosed within the framework of ephemeral life. These are the human miseries that necessitated the Great Will of Amida. The dishonest are the real reason for the existence of the Great Will.

For Master Shinran says: "If even the honest can be saved, why not the dishonest?" (The invention and the necessity of morality proves the pitiful dishonesty of humanity. It is like a palliative remedy—symptomatic, local and superficial; never the perfect therapeutic that removes the cause of illness.)

Chapter 4

There are two kinds of mercy: one, moral and limited; the other religious, transcendental, or absolute. The first is the mercy of honest people and of scholars, while the second is that of men who have faith in Supreme Joy.

The first consists in having pity, caring for, saving, and aiding materially. (Sentimental). But to save someone completely and forever is almost impossible in this world.

The second does not occupy itself directly with those things but tries to do all possible to arrive at Buddha through incessant and permanent contemplation and then, after having obtained the all-powerful Great Mercy of a Buddha, to save the entire human race. (The idea of a so-called "salvation of the world" is always illusory and injurious. Morality, moral religion, and sentimental mercy are all, like modern medicine, a Western "salvation of the world"—one that pretends to defend the individual against sickness but that accelerates the degeneration of the entire human race by interfering with natural selection. Every sentimental, moral, superficial, palliative idea is beautiful to look at, pleasant and easy to do because it deals with the "material," but it is always deceptive.)

It is impossible for us to completely "save" a pitiful being, even if we are very sincere. Mercy is infinite. How can it be an attribute of man, the lowliest of beings?

Nembutsu is the highest mercy that is permitted us.

Chapter 5

"I, Shinran, have never practiced Nembutsu while wishing for the happiness of my parents. All living beings are parents. Each of us in our turn helps one another, in one world or another. Were it by my own faculty that I did Nembutsu, I would do it for my parents. But, having once abandoned my illusory existence, and by great supernatural mercy arrived at the perfect knowledge of Buddha, I must save all that come to me through predestination. This I must do, even if I myself am sick and troubled."

Chapter 6

To strive for disciples is forbidden to followers of Nembutsu. "I, Shinran, have no disciple. If I said Nembutsu for someone through my own faculty, then he would be my disciple. But it is not through my faculty but through the Will of Amida that I do Nembutsu. How then, can anyone say he is my disciple?

"We accompany one another through Karma; we separate through Karma. To say that one cannot arrive at Buddha if he leaves one master to go towards another is not true.

"Faith is given by Amida. Does a person wish to take it back as if he himself had given it? That is impossible. When one understands the law of Great Nature, he becomes grateful to Buddha (Amida) and to his teacher."

Chapter 7

The Nembutsuist has perfect freedom. (It is the world of Supreme Consciousness.) There is no demon or evil genie that can stop him. Neither crime nor evil can lead him astray; no good action can touch him.

Chapter 8
The Nembutsu is not austere conduct; it does not result in good for the ascetic.
And if Nembutsu is not a voluntary mode of conduct, it is certainly not an austere mode of conduct. It is not a Good because one cannot do it of his own volition. That depends on the Great Will of Amida. There is in Nembutsu no impurity or influence springing from the self. It is beyond human will. For, there results no special "conduct" nor good for the Nembutsuist.

Chapter 9
Yuienbo (a disciple of Shinran) asked his teacher: "I practice Nembutsu but I never become very happy or very grateful toward Amida. No idea comes to hasten me to the land of Great Joy. Why so, Master?"
Shinran replied: "Yuien, I, too, asked that myself. But that proves to us that we are destined for the land of Great Joy. (Which is to say we are bad and dishonest.) That is why we do not become either very joyous or very happy from this Great Joy. That which prevents us from being more joyous and more happy are our sad and blind passions (that create the world of 'knowledge,' of the limited freedom of beings.) But the Great Buddha (Amida), foreseeing this, calls us 'the creatures burdened with all the desires and blind passions.' We should understand that the Great Joy is really created for beings such as us. We are happy. It is true that we have no desire to hurry toward the Great Joy (*Shunyata*), and moreover, if we are a little indisposed, we are sad and invaded by the fear of death. But, all that comes from our desires and blind passions. We are not courageous enough to go to the unknown world of the Great Joy. All that comes from our blind passions, which are very strong. When one finishes this precious life and is forced to abandon the terrestrial world, he comes to the unknown land of the Great Joy. The Great Joy impatiently awaits those who do not want to leave this sad world full of suffering as soon as

possible. If we are grateful toward Amida and joyous to go to the unknown land as soon as possible and if we hurry, we seem as strange as honest people devoid of desire and blind passion."

Chapter 10

The spirit of Nembutsu is ineffable and infinitely profound. (*Taikyoku*, *Shunyata* cannot be grasped by words.) There is no means of analyzing it. There is no possibility of understanding it perfectly. It is absolutely supernatural.

From diverse far countries, numerous seekers after truth and belief in the Great Joy, of one spirit, hastened to Kyoto and listened to the words of our master.

The followers of these disciples in their countries were innumerable. All said Nembutsu.

But, in dispute, some offered propositions foreign to those of our master. All are incomprehensible.

Chapter 11

A few, meeting a novice who was doing Nembutsu, surprised him by asking: "You do Nembutsu? But do you believe in the supernatural Great Will or do you reckon on the great power of the supernatural appellation?" Giving no explanation of these two supernatural forces and disturbing the thought of innocents is deplorable.

The appellation is the manifestation or transformation of Amida's Supreme Will. When one has deep gratitude that gratitude itself is the transformation or manifestation of the Supreme Will of Amida Buddha.

Whenever one does Nembutsu, he expresses this appellation, which will cause him to be born to the Great Joy. To believe that we are saved from an ephemeral life full of suffering by the Great Will of Amida and to see, through meditation, that to do Nembutsu is already by that Will, this will cause us to be born to the Great Joy with no impurity of thought from an illusory "ego."

When the belief in the absolutely unexplainable Great Will is given, the appellation of that saves accompanies it. The Great Will and the appellation are one. Some pedants think that good conduct distinguishes the new life in the Great Joy as opposed to bad conduct in the old life. This means they have no confidence in the Great Will, and they are counting on their own good conduct as Karma for the Great Joy. They lack the capacity to see the great incomprehensible power of the appellation. However, after having made a long detour through many intermediate steps, they arrive at the Great Joy, thanks to the Great Will and the great inexplicable power of the appellation.

[The translator (George Ohsawa) was astonished and, at first, could not reply when someone asked him: "What is the use of Nembutsu? What good does it do?"]

As it is said, the Nembutsu is a totally spontaneous appellation like the one a young child—his heart full of happiness—makes when he looks upon the face of his mother. We have no need to ask or to pray. We are right in the center of the Happiness that Great Nature offers us; we have only to busy ourselves thanking her and, even better than thanking her, to enjoy it completely. That surpasses thanksgiving. All that is necessary was prepared before man was created; we have only to make use of it. What kindness! All that we lack we lack for a reason. Everything that happens is necessary, however sad and disagreeable it may be.

The Nembutsu is an exclamation of ecstasy—tranquil and profound. It is a superlative expression of "what kindness!" All that our blind desires cause us to seek in a greater quantity than that furnished by the Great Will is injurious. It is on this point that the Orient, more or less consciously, despises modern material civilization.

[Another asked the translator, "Does Nembutsu relieve hunger?" Happiness is always confused with utility. Nembutsu does not oppose hunger; Nembutsu does not replace bread as you might wish that it did. But the Nembutsu born in hunger reveals to us the Great Will. The mechanism of hunger that protects us from death is incomprehensible by the wisdom we call physiology, but the savants believe they have explained that mechanism by a simple physical phenomenon or mechanism of the stomach. They are happy with this explanation, ignoring completely what produces the phenomenon.]

[Translator's note: Instead of trying to eliminate hunger, we should learn to enjoy it. Hunger is life.]

Chapter 12

It is unjust to say that he who does not study books or documents cannot be directed toward the new world, the Great Joy. All of the exact documents that explain the True Will say: "Have faith in the Great Will; practice Nembutsu. That is all that is necessary to become a Buddha. Indeed, what studies could be useful?"

If you cannot profoundly understand this reasoning, deepen your studies and learn the *raison d'etre* of the Great Will by a deepened ideology.

Those who study and learn from books and documents cannot understand the true *raison d'etre* of the Great Will; this is lamentable. (And, if they comprehend, it is still a literal comprehension of no value.) "Comprehension" is forbidden in the Buddhist belief. Spontaneous admiration, the innocent appellation, the ecstasy of great joy, the absolute absence of all fear are the elements of faith that distinguish it from comprehension.

He who busies himself exclusively with studies, as if Buddhism were a science, belongs to the sect of respectable men or scholars. This is the Difficult Way.

It is further said: "Those who study in order to seek worldly success, be it material or spiritual, have too many difficulties to surmount to arrive at the Great Joy."

Some Nembutsuists, in a discussion with disciples of the Difficult Way, said: "Our sect is superior; the other is inferior." Thus, they gain enemies and slander religion, and that is to insult their own religion.

We do not defend ourselves if others accuse the sect of Nembutsu of being ignorant, superficial, and contemptible. For we have learned that we who are ignorant and contemptible can be saved by belief in Nembutsu. Naturally, that appears superficial and despicable to respectable people. But to us it is sublime. Perhaps other sects are superior, but we are not qualified to join them.

Nevertheless, all the Buddhas hope that we will be saved from this illusory idea, the limiting framework of life. "We beg you then, do not hinder us." When we speak humbly in this way, who can molest us?

In addition we are taught: "When there is a dispute, evil desires are released, and we should maintain our distance."

Our master says, in the words of Shakyamuni Buddha: "Some believe in this sect, others despise it." Thus, we believe in it, but if there were no one to despise it, the words of Shakyamuni Buddha would not be true.

But that doesn't mean that "we should be insulted." Shakyamuni Buddha, foreseeing that some would insult our sect and others would believe in it, warns us in advance so that we will not be lost or deceived.

These days, do people engage in studies in order to defend themselves against insults? Is debate the purpose of their studies?

When one studies, he should gradually deepen his knowledge of the infinite grandeur of the Will of Amida. He should teach dishonest people, who, because of their bad and excessive conduct, have despaired of being saved, that there is nothing Good or Bad, Beautiful or Unbearable for the Great Will. That is what one should do.

Menacer told some people who were practicing Nembutsu that not to study was to oppose the Law. This shows a lack of faith and is misleading.

It is necessary to be prudent and not to work against the spirit of our master. A person should be especially careful not to wander without deep gratitude to Amida Buddha (into the petty ego world of knowledge).

Chapter 13

It is said that "to rely too much on the Great Will of Amida and not to fear evil is also an evil and prevents one from arriving at the Great Joy." But this is a lack of faith in the Great Will and is still ignorance of the Karma of good and evil.

To have the intent to do Good is by Karma and to have the intent to do Evil is also Karma.

Our master says: "Even a crime as light as a speck of dust on a hair of a rabbit cannot be committed except by Karma." (This is moral determinism.)

One day the master Shinran said to his disciple Yuien: "Yuien, do you believe what I tell you?"

"With great pleasure," replied Yuien very respectfully.

"Well then, you will not disobey if I tell you to do something."

The disciple affirmed very respectfully.

"Good. Go out and kill a thousand men, and you will be assured of the Great Joy," said Shinran.

"If it is your order, but I do not believe myself capable of killing even one person," replied Yuien.

"Why then have you promised to do as I say?"

"Know well that a man does only what pleases him. If it were pleasant for you, you would kill a thousand men to be able to enter into the Great Joy. But you cannot kill even one person because your Karma will not permit you. It is not through your good will that you will not kill. You will kill hundreds or thousands of men without knowing it or wanting it.

"To believe ourselves capable of judging good and evil is complete ignorance of the Great Will." He explained himself in this way:

There was a man obsessed with a pitiful idea: "The Great Will saves him who does evil;" and he committed the evils of his choice in order to enter into the Land of the Great Joy. Having heard of this, Master Shinran wrote very simply to this man: "If you have medicine, you do not have to drink poison." That doesn't mean, however, that evil is an obstacle on the road to the Great Joy.

If obedience to commandments and the observance of rules are the only means of believing in the Great Will, how can we save ourselves from the limitation of ephemeral life? When we, whose actions are so pitiful and unimportant, find the Great Will, we become proud of our existence.

One can never commit a single wrong deed except through Karma.

Fishing or hunting in order to earn a living is similar to the work of a merchant or farmer who cultivates the fields. One does all that Karma obliges him to do.

These days, some people, pretending to have a deep knowledge of the Great Joy, believe that "respectable people" alone can do Nembutsu. Or they put on the walls of the lecture halls: "Entrance is forbidden to him who does such and such a thing . . ." They pretend to be honest while hiding the most profound ignorance.

If one does evil because of excessive reliance on the Great Will, it is also through Karma.

To abandon all conventional ideology, to trust and allow Karma to do all, be it Good or Evil, and to have complete confidence in the Great Will—that is the Easy Way.

It is said in "Yuisinshyo" that "it is pitiful to see people who say they have committed too many sins to be saved and who voluntarily enclose themselves in an abyss of despair. They do not know how great is the supernatural power of the Great Will."

Reliance in the Great Will is even indispensable for faith in the Easy Way.

If, after having abandoned passion and desire, one could have faith in the Great Will, it would be very just. But if one abandoned all passion and desire, one would already be a Buddha. Faith in the Great Will is useless for a Buddha (because his will is the Great Will. There is no separation).

Those who reproach others for being too reliant on the Great Will are also saddled with blind passions and desires and, hence, are themselves relying on the Great Will.

"What is the Evil that is called the reliance on the Great Will?"

"What is the Evil that is not reliance? How naive!"

[Translator's comments: It is sad to hear some people say that they are satisfied with themselves because they are not proud. In reality, they are proud of their humility. In the same way, those who are content at having done no wrong are completely unaware that their morals are a convenience. To be proud of what doesn't exist except in imagination is dangerous and criminal.

In the same way, all those who think themselves honest, humble, charitable, and fraternal are to be pitied.

To behave humbly, to do a good deed, to be thankful a thousand times over in words or deeds, and to be happy with that is considered to be insignificant in Buddhism. We do good when it pleases us to do so.

Let us give a dime to a beggar. If he not only doesn't thank us, but on the other hand, insults us for the smallness of the gift, we are angry because we expected thanks. To tell the truth, this was a transaction not a good deed. Unconsciously, we had the intention of buying an agreeable feeling for a dime. Lacking a dime or in different circumstances, we would give nothing.

All this good conduct is too conspicuous and conditional, never an Absolute Good Will. It is sentimental, superficial, capricious, and more or less mixed with vanity and fantasy. It is conditioned and limited. It is something that anyone could do under the same conditions. If it were Absolute Will, it would be necessary for you to give all you possess without ulterior motives, even your blood or your life. If the beggar accepted your offer, you should, through him, very profoundly thank the Great Will for his existence, for your existence, and for what you have given him.

According to Buddhist belief, sentimentalism is useless and injurious, for it is individualism teaching us to be moral while indulging in self-love.

The people are too simple to understand the true significance of the phrase "know thyself." They can observe this philosophy under convenient conditions, but at the same time, they begin to think themselves honest and become proud of their morals. There is the danger. The people are unaware that the necessity of such a morality has its origin in our profound dishonesty, which is impossible to completely uproot.]

Chapter 14

It is said that one can erase numerous sins through one Nembutsu. This is to say that the most dishonest person, instructed in the Great Will by a person knowing the Law, can do Nembutsu for the first time at the last moment of his life and redeem his numerous sins. If he repeats Nembutsu ten times, he can even redeem ten times as many sins. This is simply to show the insignificance of our ten great evils and five great sins in comparison to the great power of Nembutsu. It is rudimentary instruction, more for beginners or for simplistic people than for us. Once illuminated by the Light of Amida, the intention to do Nembutsu comes to us when solid and sublime belief is established. We are ephemeral life, Amida transforms all our blind desires and passions into true happiness—perfect, eternal, and invariable. Without this Great Will, it is impossible to save ourselves from the narrow framework of life. For we believe that all Nembutsu that we do during our life is to repay the Great Gratitude of Amida. To believe that we redeem our sins with every Nembutsu is to rely on our imaginative capacity to shape our own conduct, to redeem our sins with that conduct, and to go to the Great Joy.

All that we do does not go beyond the framework of ephemeral life. Let us do Nembutsu unceasingly until the last breath in order to enter into the Great Joy. However, we are governed by supernatural Karma, and we do not know if, though accident or illness, we may not end our lives unable to do Nembutsu. In this case, what should we do to redeem our mistakes? Is it impossible to arrive at the Great Joy without completely redeeming them all?

If we believe that the Great Will abandons no one, we understand that we are saved within the Great Joy even though, after a life full of sins, we do not do Nembutsu. If you can continue to do Nembutsu, make it stronger and stronger as you approach the last moment until you obtain true solid belief. Do this to repay the Great Gratitude of Amida.

To strive to redeem mistakes belongs to the narrow and egoistical mentality of the Difficult Way. It corresponds to the spirit of respectable people and is useless for us Nembutsuists of the Easy Way.

Chapter 15

To arrive at the Great Joy through mastery of passion and desire is very difficult for us. To live the life of a Buddha with the physical body is the *raison d'etre* of the Sacred Shingon Sect and the consequence of its three conducts of austerity. The suppression of desires and passion (of five physical categories and one spiritual category) is the principle of the Hokké Sect and the glory of its four spiritual forms of behavior. All are forms of behavior corresponding to the Difficult Way of respectable and highly placed people—the perfecting of saintly comprehension.

To be saved in the other world (after death) is the principle of the Easy Way, the True Sect of the Great Joy. It is the road of belief for lowly people such as us, where the Law does not distinguish good from evil. (Shinran strove to give us complete knowledge of our fleeting, insignificant existence, or our absolute ignorance, the knowledge of ignorance, the "consciousness" of *Shunyata*.)

It is difficult to destroy all desires and passions in this world. Consequently, the ascetics of Hokké and Shingon do not disdain praying for future life.

We don't have good conduct or wisdom, but we are embarked on the great ship "Great Will of Amida" that transports us across the sad ocean of life and death. We will arrive on the shore of the Great Joy where we will look in wonder at the moon, "consciousness." Cleared of all desire and passion, it will illuminate us with an infinite and penetrating light that shines unimpeded in every direction, saving us all. That signals our arrival into the Great Joy.

Whoever enters into the Great Joy in this life is a Shakyamuni Buddha who can transform himself into whatever he wants, who possesses the 32 gracious points of physiognomy and 80 physical superiorities, who teaches the Law and who saves the world. That is the attainment of saintly comprehension in the world.

It is said in the hymn "Wasan": "When solid faith is obtained, one is saved forever; there is no need to be tormented by the detour through the six intermediate steps; one is outside of this narrow framework of life." This is often misunderstood; it is lamentable.

"The True Sect of the Great Joy teaches us to believe in the Great Will in this world and to enter into the Great Joy in the next world," said the Master Shinran.

Chapter 16

It is said: "When the Nembutsuists become angry and commit evils or argue brashly without conscience with friends, they should always make a conversion." Does that mean that they try to suppress evil and do good?

For the Nembutsuists, there is only one conversion. When the stranger to the Great Will, having been instructed by the wisdom of Amida, learns that he cannot attain the Great Peace by the method he has practiced up until that time, he abandons it and takes on the belief in the Great Will. That is the only conversion.

If a person had to do conversion in respect to all action, morning and night, he would die without perfecting the conversion or arriving at a peaceable mentality. Theoretically, the Great Will would be incapable of saving him.

In saying, "I believe in the Great Will," one believes at the bottom of his heart that "even thought the Great Will is true and supernatural, it will be the honest people that will be saved." One doubts the Great Will. One lacks faith in it and must make a detour through intermediate steps. That is lamentable.

Once faith is established, it is Amida that arranges all that is necessary to attain Great Joy. It isn't our doing at all.

Willing or not, once faith is established in the depth of the great omnipotent power of the Great Will, even the dishonest person, of necessity, becomes persevering and consequently tranquil and joyous.

In any case, let us not strive to pretend to be wise in order to attain the Great Joy, but let us have absolute and unceasing confidence in the gratitude of the Great Will. Then one can practice Nembutsu involuntarily. It comes spontaneously. That which one does with no ulterior motive is inspired by the Great Will. *Shunyata*, the philosophy of Shinran, is the philosophy of spontaneity.

Some people say that they concern themselves exclusively with spontaneity as if they were the only ones to do so. How pitiful.

Chapter 17

It is said that those who descend through intermediate steps finally fall into Hell. However, there is no sacred document that confirms this. It is unfortunate that scholars say such things. How do they interpret the just books and exact documents?

It is said, in fact, that "the ascetics that lack faith, doubt the Great Will, and fall into Hendi (an intermediate step), redeem their errors, and finally attain Great Joy."

As there are few people that have deep faith, many are sent to intermediate stages. To say that these people are abandoned to Hell is to blaspheme Amida.

Chapter 18

To say that the value or quantity of an offering distinguishes the new Buddha-like life in the Great Joy is not true. The new life, the life of Buddha, is just the same. If one describes the greatness of size of Master Buddha of the Great Joy, it is only a pious artifice.

Once the knowledge of the Great Will is established, form is no longer important; the coloring—blue, yellow, red, white or black— is unimportant because one is considering all existence from the point of view of Inner Nature. (See the chapter on Chinese Science in the Unique Principle and *Maha Prajna Paramita Hridaya Sutra,* which follows.) There is no need to distinguish or define an illusory grandeur.

It is said that one sees the illusion of Buddha while practicing meditation. It could probably be said that one will see the great illusion of Buddha in a long contemplation and a small illusion in a shorter contemplation. Perhaps it is through this reasoning that one deceives himself into thinking that the offering distinguishes the new life. This may also be the reasoning behind *danaparamita* (an action that consists of offering all you possess). If one lacks faith, all alms and offerings lose significance. If one believes deeply in the

Great Will, he will correspond to the *raison d'etre* of the Great Will without offering a penny or even a scrap of paper.

Or possibly, that (the offering distinguishes the new life . . . etc.) is the word of one who wants to utilize Buddhism for his own purposes.

All of the misunderstandings depend on faith. The Master Shinran often said that he hadn't many disciples who were as firm in their faith as the disciples who surrounded the Master Honen.

One day he was discussing this with friends. "My faith is equal to that of our master, Honen."

The disciples, among them Seikanbo and Nembutsu, objected. "How can the faith of Shinran be the equal of our master's faith?" Shinran explained by saying, "If I said that my "knowledge" is equal to the infinite wisdom of our master, that would be false. But I am saying that my faith in the Great Joy (the "consciousness" of *Shunyata*) is absolutely similar to that of our master."

"That is impossible," said the others.

Finally, they presented themselves to the Master Honen and asked him to judge.

Master Honen said, "My faith is given by Amida; Shinran's faith is also given by Amida. There is no difference between them. If anyone has a different belief than mine, he will never arrive at the Great Joy where I, Genku, have arrived."

Let it be known that in those times, even among Nembutsuists, there were some who misunderstood faith.

I repeat this, even though it may be useless. Already old and trembling like the last leaf on the tree, I will continue to explain what I heard from my master to my friends. But I fear there will be a throng of misunderstandings and disorders when my eyes are closed forever. For that reason, I am writing these lines.

If you are led astray by these people, look carefully into the books and documents that our master recommended to us.

Generally speaking, there is, in education, both truth and pious artifice. Grasp the truth and don't bother yourself with provisional means. That is the wish of our master. Do not do superficial reading.

I will add a few lines from precious documents to serve you as a guide. The master said: "I have long contemplated and I have at last understood that the Eternal Will of Amida was established completely for me and for me alone, in order to save me from Karma. What generosity!" This is similar to the words of Zendo. He said: "That I might know! I am a mediocre man, dishonest and despicable who drifts around like the eddies in a stream, unable to go beyond this life of suffering."

The Master Shinran said again: "I do not know Good or Evil. If I could know all the Good that Amida knows, I could then say that I know Good. If I could know all the Evil that Amida condemns, I could say I know Evil. But, in reality, I am a mediocre man. What do I know? I know nothing."

"In this fleeting, fragile world, all is false and ephemeral. There is no truth. Only Nembutsu is true."

One of the most foolish things one can do is to insist on something that is foreign to the words of our master in teaching Nembutsu.

Understand this profoundly, I beg you.

What I say here has no value because I know nothing of the profound truth of the books nor of the teaching of the sacred documents. Excuse me. I am simply writing a few of the words of our master that my memory dictates to me. It is sad to go to Hendi instead of going directly to the Great Joy, even if one has learned Nembutsu.

My eyes are wet with tears; I write these lines, hoping that all my friends are united in the unique belief. I call them "Tannishyo" (Regret for Foreign Belief). Do not show them to others who believe in knowledge, technique, and superiority of ego.

It was under the reign of the Emperor Gotobain (12th century) that Honen preached the True Sect of Nembutsu of the Great Will, the Easy Way.

Some of his disciples were very passionate. Their adversaries, the monks of Kohoku-ji of Nara, the Village of the South, took advantage of that to impede the spread of their doctrine. They had Honen and his disciples arrested and condemned for their calumnies.

This was the result:

Honen, at the age of 76, was exiled to Hakata-de-Tosa on the island of Shikoku, under the accursed name of Hujii-Motohiko.

Shinran, age 35, was exiled to Echigo under the accursed name of Hujii-Zenshin.

Zyomon-bo was exiled to Bingo; Chosei-Zenko-bo to Hoki; Kokaku-bo to Izu; Gyoku-Hohan-bo to Sado; Kazei-Zyogaku-bo and Zenaku-bo were entrusted to the care of Bishop Zendai, thanks to the generosity of the latter.

Seii-Zenshaku-bo was condemned to death as well as Seigan-bo, Zyuren-bo, and Anraku-bo.

All of these sentences were signed by Nii-Hoin-Takanaga, the governor.

Shinran was deprived of his Buddhist rank and was given a lay name. He was neither a monk nor a layman because his head was shaved according to Buddhist custom. After that he called himself "Toku" (Shaved Head) or "Gutoku" (Ignorant Shaved Head, Mediocre Man).

Appendix 2

The Secret of the Perfect Consciousness
(Maha Prajna Paramita Hridaya Sutra)

[Translator's note: This sutra is the supreme secret of the philosophy of Buddhism. If one understood this secret, one would have no need to study all the numerous books concerning Buddhism. Even with knowledge of all these meaningless books, one is profane in Buddhism if he does not understand it. It is very difficult to decipher. Few persons have understood it.]

Vocabulary

Shunyata: *Taikyoku*, Ether-Universe, True Universe, or Tao. See the "Theory of Being" and the "Theory of Knowledge of the Far-East," Part 2.

Perfect Consciousness: The consciousness that recognizes the world of beings in the Universe of *Shunyata*.

Avalokiteshvara Bodhisattva: Buddha contemplating the physical and spiritual world at his will, personifying the Perfect Consciousness.

Shariputra: Well-known disciple of Shakyamuni, representing the "instinct-intuition" (always according to the "Theory of Being" and the "Theory of Knowledge of the Far-East").

Dharma: All existence in *Shunyata*, the True Universe, simultaneously exterior and intimate. That is, all beings, intimate nature, and the law that unifies them.

Skandha: Five aggregates which form the world. The world is considered in Buddhist philosophy as resulting from five aggregates: physical phenomena, the sensation that sees them, thought that is born from sensation, wishes (desires) that detach themselves from thought, and the knowledge that one obtains from these last ones mentioned.

Maha Prajna Paramita Hridaya Sutra: (Maka Hannya Hara Mita Shin Gyo—Japanese pronunciation)
Avalokiteshvara-Bodhisattva, having explained at length to Shariputra the secret of the Perfect Consciousness that saves the world from all sufferings, showed that Skandha is completely of *Shunyata*. He concluded:

Shariputra, the physical phenomena are therefore of *Shunyata*. *Shunyata* expresses itself in phenomena. Phenomena are therefore *Shunyata. Shunyata* is phenomena. Again the sensations, the thought, the wishes, and the knowledge are nothing other than *Shunyata*.

Shariputra, all Dharma is a property of *Shunyata*. He is not born nor does he disappear. He cannot be invalidated nor purified; he does not increase or diminish. There is not in the true universe any phenomenon or sensation or thought or desire of knowledge. Sight, hearing, smell, taste, body and mind—all are useless. Visual phenomena, sounds and words, odor, tastes, sensations, and ethics do not exist. From the visual world to the ethical and spiritual world, nothing exists any longer.

In *Shunyata,* there is no obscurity. At the same time, there is no end to obscurity. There is neither aging nor death; at the same time, no end to it. It is, therefore, impossible for suffering to exist in *Shunyata*, nor causes, wishes, Nirvana, nor the way to arrive there. Neither does knowing nor not knowing because there is no having.

A Bodhisattva who has the Perfect Consciousness is free of all doubt and of all hesitation. He has no fear because he has no doubt or hesitation. He is therefore liberated from all blind desires and all dreams and attains Nirvana.

All the Buddhas of the past, present, and future arrive at the Supreme Consciousness of *Shunyata* by the Perfect Consciousness.

We have hence understood that the secret of the Perfect Consciousness is the great divine secret, that it is the secret Unique and

Supreme, that it suppresses all suffering. It is true. It is not false. Therefore, we meditate and adore the secret as Mantra, of the Perfect Consciousness.

All arrive
at the banks, beyond,
all gather together
by the consciousness
perfect and adorable

George Rodenbach

I still do not know enough of the philosophical, scientific and literary authors to know which are those to whom the spirit is the closest by their conception of the universe and of the Oriental spirit. I have only met by chance a poet, George Rodenbach, whose entire work seems to attach itself to a simple idea very similar to that of the consciousness of being, such as we have studied. Especially in his poem "Mental Aquarium," we see written *Taikyoku*, *Shunyata*, True Universe, immobile and mobile, transparent and opaque, outside of time and of space—so much so that one can translate by the words unknown qualities equal to the physical life.

> The aquarium is so bluish, so lunar;
> Window of infinity opening upon what garden?
> Mirror of eternity of which the sky is the reflector.
> To what recoil is she going to extend
> Her azure, ventilated by shutters of gold? In this
> opaque basin where their sort is exiled,
> Place which is no longer life and is not death.
> The aquarium does not at first seem alive,
> Uninhabited, like a mirror in a convent;
> Crepuscule where always a mist is formed; it sleeps
> so palely that one would believe it dead and that
> The black reflections which come and go
> are only shadows without aim on the death bed
> and furtive games of night light on the ceiling.

Biography of George Ohsawa

Year   Age

1893   Sakurazawa Nyoichi was born in Kyoto, Japan, on October 18.

1902   9   His mother died when she was thirty. His father disappeared and he had to take care of his younger brother and sister.

1908   15   He developed Tuberculosis of the lung and intestine. He suffered from many other diseases.

1912   19   He reestablished his health by the diet taught by Dr. Sagen Ishizuka. He graduated from the First Commercial High School in Kyoto. He was employed by the Takinami Company in Kobe as a messenger boy and attended Kobe French School.

1914   21   Graduated from the French School but lost the job when the company closed the business because of the beginning of World War I. He was employed by Wormth Steamship Co., England, as a purser on the Manei Maru. He went to Europe for the first time during World War I.

1915   22   Employed by Nakagiri Trading Co. in Kobe as a manager.

1917 24 Founded Kumasawa Trading Co. in Kobe as a branch of Kumasawa Co., which was a wholesale textile company. He was chosen as manager. Traveled to Europe every other year. He started a movement for the reformation of the Japanese language through the publication of the magazine *Yomigaeri*.

1920 27 He brought the first broadcasting radio transmitter and receiver from France to Japan. Through his own invention, he improved on existing movie and still cameras.

1925 31 The control of the company was taken over by the investors. This event made him decide to quit business. He moved to Tokyo and started his life work by joining the Macrobiotic Association and Japanese Language Association. (Shokuyo-Kai and Nippon Romaji Association.)

1927 34 Elected director of the Shokuyo-Kai and was editor of the magazine Shokuyo, which means Macrobiotic.

1928 35 Held the first Macrobiotic summer camp in Hokkaido. Published five volumes of the "Macrobiotic Discourse" and a biography of Sagen Ishizuka.

1929 36 Visited Paris via the Siberian Railway without any financial support and then published *Unique Principle* in French (Vrin Co., Paris).

1930 37 Although living a very poor life in Paris, he managed to study at both the Sorbonne University and the Pasteur Institute. He taught Oriental medicine, Acupuncture, flower arrangement, Judo, and Haiku to the French people and published two books, *The Oriental Medicine* (Hippocrates Publishers) and *Book of Flowers* (Vrin Co.)

1935 42 Returned to Japan and advised Generals S. Araki and Y. Iimori not to make war against Western Powers.

1937 44 Elected president of the Shokuyo-Kai (Macrobiotic Association). The subscribers of the *Shokuyo* had by then reached ten thousand. He published *Man the Unknown* written by Alexis Carrel.

1939 46 Published a book called *Making Westerners Enemies*, which expressed such strong anti-militarism that it caused heavy antagonism among the military and super patriots of Japan. He could not safely stay in Japan under these conditions. In order to escape these dangers from the Nationalists, he became a health consultant for the Emperor's family and other nobles. He published *A New Dietetic Cure*, which sold millions of copies. He resigned from the Shokuyo-Kai.

1940 47 He founded the Unique Principle Institute in Ohtsu, Kyoto, where he taught the Unique Principle instead of how to cure diseases.

1941 48 He published 100,000 copies of "The Health Front of the World," which warned the Japanese government leaders that they would destroy Japan and bring confusion to the country similar to that during the French Revolution. He also predicted that they would be shot. His prophecy was realized four years later at the end of the war. However, his warning was so strong that there was grave danger of his assassination.

He published the book *One Who Wins Last and Eternally* in which he made the prophecy that England would abandon India and that Gandhi would be assassinated. This prophecy came true in five years.

The book *Making Westerners Enemies: Who Will Destroy Japan* was purged by the Japanese government. 2000 books were burned.

1942   49   He published the books *Newer Nutrition, The History of China, An Expedition in the Bacterial World, A Primitive Mentality and Japanese Mentality,* and *A Study of Sun Tsu and Other Strategies.* At that time, pressure from the military government increased daily. He was tortured by the military police for six months.

1944   51   In July, he predicted that Japan would be defeated. Japan surrendered the next year. To all students who were at the front, he sent telegrams that read: "You should eat carefully and be the last winner." Published two anti-war and anti-militaristic books, *An Eternal Child—Anatole France* and *How to Change Heart.* In November, he tried to reach Moscow through Manchuria in order to ask Russia to be a mediator of World War II. En route, he was chased by the military police and forced to change his plan. He escaped capture, however, and returned to Japan to plan another attempt.

1945   52   On January 25, he was captured in his hide-out and jailed under conditions in which the temperature went as low as 20 degrees below zero (centigrade). After three months of such treatment, he became extremely weak, lost 80 percent of his eyesight, and almost died.

At the end of June, he was suddenly released with the stipulation that he would not bring a law suit against the government.

In July, he attempted a *coup d'etat* with Generals Iimori and Fujimori but was captured again at a secret meeting and was jailed in Kofu and subsequently transferred to prison in Nagasaki. Kofu was bombed completely after he was moved. In August, Japan surrendered. In September, he was released by the order of General Mac Arthur, just before the execution of his death sentence. He wrote a letter appealing to MacArthur, advising him to diminish the military and secret police of the Japanese government. The advice was taken and those systems were abolished. In October, he published the book *Why Did Japan Fail?* In December, he started the True Life COOP in Tokyo and the monthly magazine *Compas*.

1946 53 Started seminars in Yokohama on the biological and educational revolution of man.

1947 54 Joined United World Federalists Organization.

1948 55 He started a Macrobiotic Study House (Called Maison Ignoramus) in Hiyoshi, Tokyo, which moved soon to Yoyogi-Nishihara. Published the volume *Book of Judo* in French.

1949 56 He was active in the World Government movement in various cities. His world government movement was based on the idea that world peace is only possible when individuals are able to establish their own health and happiness through biological and physiological improvement.

1950 57 He met Norman Cousins who was visiting Hiroshima to attend a peace movement. Translated and published *Meeting East and West* written by F.S.C. Northrop in Japanese.

1952 59   Published *Eternal Boy—A Biography of Benjamin Franklin* in Japan.

1953 60   Left Japan for India to teach Macrobiotics to the world.

1954 61   Founded Indo-Japan Cultural Center in India. Wrote an open letter to Mao Tse-Tung in which he advised him on his health and on the policy of China from the standpoint of Macrobiotics.

1955 62   In June, he left India and went to Africa by boat. Arrived at Lambarene, Gabon on October 29. He began teaching Macrobiotics to the black people.

1956 62   From January 25, he suffered from tropical ulcers, a disease which is almost always fatal. This was cured in about ten days by the Macrobiotic diet. (Please read *Cancer and the Philosophy of the Far East.*) He advised Dr. Schweitzer to adopt the Macrobiotic diet for his patients. Dr. Schweitzer disagreed, and then Ohsawa left Lambarene. On February 29, he arrived in Paris, where 25 years previously he had planted the seeds of Oriental culture.

1956 63   He lectured day and night on Macrobiotics in Belgium, Switzerland, Germany, Sweden, Italy, and England. A Macrobiotic factory (Lima) was soon started in Belgium, and Macrobiotic stores and restaurants began all over Europe.

1957 64   He started the publication of the French magazine *Yin and Yang*, which is still continuing.

1958 65   *Oriental Medicine* and *Jack and Mitie* were published in French.

1959 66   He visited the United States for the first time in December of this year.

1960 67   In New York, he published the book *Zen Macrobiotics* in English by mimeograph. In January, he began ten daily seminars for Americans at the Buddhist Academy, NYC. In February and March, additional seminars were held. He returned to Europe in April but flew back to America to attend the First American Summer Camp in Long Island, New York, which was held from July to August. He gave lectures everyday for two months. The first American Macrobiotic magazine *Macrobiotic News* was started in New York. This is now continuing as *Macrobiotics Today* (published by the George Ohsawa Macrobiotic Foundation in Chico, California).

1961 68   The *Philosophy of Oriental Medicine* was published in English, which he wrote and originally published in Japan. The second American Summer Camp was held at Wortzboro, New York in July and August with great success.

1962 69   Some of his students started the first American Macrobiotic food manufacturing and distributing company in Chico. His summer camp in France that year was a great success.

1963 70   *Atomic Age* was published in French. He flew to the U.S. again and gave lectures with other Japanese lecturers in New York City, Boston, and California Summer Camps.

On August 18, his prediction that John F. Kennedy would experience great danger was published by the New York Herald Tribune. This prediction was realized the next year with the death of President Kennedy.

1964   71   He and his disciples succeeded in an atomic transmuta-
tion experiment (Na-K) on July 21. Shortly afterward,
he lectured at the Big Sur Summer Camp in California.

1965   72   He started to organize a spiritual olympic in Japan. *You
are All Sanpaku* was published in English and a French
translation of *The Book of Cancer* was published in
France. He flew to America and gave lectures at Mayoro
Lodge near Pulga, California. He gave lectures in five
places in Europe and America that year on a tour that
covered 20,000 miles.

1966   73   On April 24 at 5:30 p.m., he left this world eternally.
The cause of his death was diagnosed as a heart attack
by his doctors. "Education of the Will" was his last arti-
cle. The spiritual olympic originated by him was held in
Japan in July and August and was attended by over one
hundred Macrobiotic people from all over the world.

Other Books from the
George Ohsawa Macrobiotic Foundation

Acid Alkaline Companion - Carl Ferré; 2009; 121 pp; $15.00

Acid and Alkaline - Herman Aihara; 1986; 121 pp; $9.95

As Easy As 1, 2, 3 - Pamela Henkel and Lee Koch; 1990; 176 pp; $6.95

Basic Macrobiotic Cooking, 20th Anniversary Edition - Julia Ferré; 2007; 275 pp; $17.95

Basic Macrobiotics - Herman Aihara; 1998; 198 pp; $17.95

Book of Judo - George Ohsawa; 1990; 150 pp; $14.95

Calendar Cookbook - Cornellia Aihara; 1979; 160 pp; $24.95

Cancer and the Philosophy of the Far East - George Ohsawa; 1981; 165 pp; $14.95

Cooking with Rachel - Rachel Albert; 1989; 328 pp; $12.95

Essential Ohsawa - George Ohsawa, edited by Carl Ferré; 1994; 238 pp; $12.95

French Meadows Cookbook - Julia Ferré; 2008; 275 pp; $17.00

Macrobiotics: An Invitation to Health and Happiness - George Ohsawa; 1971; 128 pp; $11.95

Naturally Healthy Gourmet - Margaret Lawson with Tom Monte; 1994; 232 pp; $14.95

Philosophy of Oriental Medicine - George Ohsawa; 1991; 153 pp; $14.95

Pocket Guide to Macrobiotics - Carl Ferré; 1997; 128 pp; $6.95

Zen Cookery - G.O.M.F.; 1985; 140 pp; $17.00

Zen Macrobiotics, Unabridged Edition - George Ohsawa, edited by Carl Ferré; 1995; 206 pp; $9.95

A complete selection of macrobiotic books is available from the George Ohsawa Macrobiotic Foundation, P.O. Box 3998, Chico, California 95965; 530-566-9765. Order toll free: (800) 232-2372. Or, see *www.ohsawamacrobiotics.com* for all books and PDF downloads of many books.

Printed in Great Britain
by Amazon

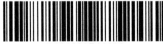